Coronavirus, Class and Mutual Aid
in the United Kingdom

John Preston • Rhiannon Firth

Coronavirus, Class and Mutual Aid in the United Kingdom

palgrave
macmillan

John Preston
Department of Sociology
University of Essex
Colchester, UK

Rhiannon Firth
Department of Sociology
University of Essex
Colchester, UK

ISBN 978-3-030-57713-1   ISBN 978-3-030-57714-8   (eBook)
https://doi.org/10.1007/978-3-030-57714-8

Cover illustration: © Boris SV / Getty images

This Palgrave Macmillan imprint is published by the registered company Springer Nature Switzerland AG.
The registered company address is: Gewerbestrasse 11, 6330 Cham, Switzerland

Contents

About the Authors

John Preston is Professor of Sociology at the University of Essex. He works on social inequalities and how they are produced and reinforced in disasters and emergencies. He is the author of several books on disaster preparedness including *Grenfell Tower: Preparedness, Race and Disaster Capitalism* (2019).

Rhiannon Firth is Senior Research Officer in Sociology at the University of Essex. She works on anarchist utopias, anti-authoritarian social movements and prefigurative politics. She is the author of the book *Utopian Politics* (2012) and is writing a second sole-authored book on *Disaster Anarchism* (under contract).

1

Introduction

John Preston and Rhiannon Firth

Capitalism has been described as akin to the destruction of space by time or time-space compression (Harvey 2000). In the world of 1918 news of pandemic influenza was slow to spread and there were areas of the world that did not know, until reasonably late in the pandemic, that there was a disaster on a global scale. Substantive international travel was relatively rare. Although the ruling class had always indulged in global 'grand tours' ships and rail provided the means of mass transit across the globe. The 'Spanish Flu' of 1918 was xenophobically and regionally named but had a truly global spread. COVID-19, similarly, is also a pandemic disease which spread globally through mass world transit but where information on the pandemic is also shared quickly through social media and constantly breaking news. Air travel brings about the rapid transit of capitalists, tourists and workers around the world and the virus spreads quickly between countries. Leisure is commodified on a mass scale so that people are brought together in giant stadia for football matches, racing events or rock concerts. Work requires mass transit systems so that collectivised workforces can be brought in and out of cities and towns sharing air and facilities. The unemployed are required to show up to sign on for benefits *en-masse*. Despite the increased efficiency of (underfunded) public health

© The Author(s) 2020
J. Preston, R. Firth, *Coronavirus, Class and Mutual Aid in the United Kingdom*,
https://doi.org/10.1007/978-3-030-57714-8_1

systems the virus continues to spread globally, accelerated by the creation and maintenance of the capitalist world market. The shrinking of the world market through communication and mass transit, concentration of working-class populations and destruction of national borders as described in the *Communist Manifesto* (Marx and Engels 2002) also produce connected 'human factories' for viral production.

Worldwide pandemics are only one cause of human death on a mass scale. The impacts of global poverty and immiseration, imperialist wars and environmental devastation are much more effective human and planetary killers. However, global pandemics can have massive and unequally distributed impacts on mortality and health. The possible source of the current COVID-19 epidemic has been identified as arising from profitable 'wet markets' (where live animals are sold) in Wuhan, China, where the virus jumped from animal (possibly a bat or pangolin) to human infection. This leap in infection cross-species has been common for other sources of illness which begin as zoonotic and then progressed to human to human transmission. In the case of this particular virus that jump occurred quickly and efficiently. As a coronavirus, SARS-CoV-2, the virus that causes the disease COVID-19, has much in common with other viruses of this type such as SARS and MERS. SARS-CoV-2 causes respiratory infections and ultimately organ failure. It spreads primarily through respiratory droplets (breath, coughs and sneezes). There is evidence that the virus that leads to COVID-19 can exist on hard surfaces for some time, particularly plastics, which led to concerns as to whether the virus can also exist on banknotes and packaging. As SARS-CoV-2 is a newly discovered virus not much is known about the virus' epidemiology other than that it is highly infectious even (perhaps a matter of weeks) before symptoms begin to appear. There seems to be a range of illnesses that might occur from the barely noticeable, through the mild (cough, high temperature, sore throat) to the serious (difficulty breathing, destruction of lung tissue and multiple organ failure) and fatal. Primarily older people and those with pre-existing conditions are impacted by the virus which has a high mortality rate that exponentially increases with age. Death and serious illness in the UK from the virus are more likely in working class, black/Asian groups and those in areas of economic deprivation. The virus is potentially in the 'sweet spot' where a series of waves of global outbreaks amounting to 1918 proportions is theoretically possible and appears to be an increasingly realistic prospect. If a virus 'burns' too quickly through human bodies then the chances of spread are reduced. Ebola, for example, where the death and incapacity rate is high and devastating, has not become a global pandemic partly because victims die quickly before they can spread the virus. The transmission route for Ebola is also not as direct as that of viruses that can spread by respiratory means. Influenza (the flu) spreads more easily as victims are not incapacitated immediately and due to vaccines and other public measures the death rate is not high. Less is currently known about transmission of COVID-19 but it seems likely that those infected can spread the disease without even being aware that they have it as it spreads easily through coughs, sneezes and surfaces. Unlike influenza there is no cure for COVID-19 and any antibodies that are likely to develop might only offer short-term protection against the illness. Public health systems, many of which are already impoverished by austerity, are quickly overwhelmed by the spread of the disease as many of those infected will require intensive care beds or complex forms of treatment. Because of its virulence, COVID-19 has taken hold in various countries. Infections in China accelerated rapidly after the reporting of the first cases in December 2019 and throughout the first few months of 2020 there were outbreaks of COVID-19 in nearly every country with initial 'hot spots' in South Korea and Italy. By early March every country, particularly in Europe and North America, was impacted. In the United Kingdom (UK) cases are growing at an exponential rate with the first death in the UK reported on 5th March 2020 accelerating so that by 12th of May there were 32,065 official deaths in the UK although there are concerns that this figure is an under-estimate and at the time of writing 'excess deaths' in the UK are estimated at over 55,000. The UK is likely to have one of the highest death rates in the world by the end of the pandemic.

This book considers the COVID-19 pandemic through a case study of how the UK government is currently preparing the population at the outset of the outbreak in 2020 and reflections on how this might produce new solutions outside of the market or the state. The framework employed is influenced by Marxism, Anarchism, class theory, social movement analysis and critical analysis of preparedness.

In Chap. 2 we consider how COVID-19 is being deployed as an element of a continuing class struggle between capital and labour. The argument is that capitalism creates and maintains capital at a multitude of scales, including the viral, and that COVID-19 as a virus and its material and discursive consequences are an active part of capital accumulation, continuing class struggle and class formation. COVID-19 operates as an element of class struggle in terms of a 'war from above' of the ruling class in terms of its use as a 'force of nature' in eugenics and against surplus populations, in creating new commodities and markets and as a justification for the deployment of an increasingly authoritarian RSA (Repressive State Apparatus) to ensure that workers continue to labour under increasingly dangerous conditions. Chapter 3 considers the UK's preparedness plans as using 'class practices' which are tacitly designed to disadvantage and divide the working class in favour of elements of the middle class and examines the behavioural science underpinning pandemic preparedness for COVID-19 uncovering its classed assumptions in terms of how distinctions, markets and altruism operate. It also considers how social isolation and quarantine function as a classed practice and how government policies make assumptions concerning housing, social practices and resources as a form of violence against the working class. Chapter 4 concludes the book by looking at alternatives to neo-liberal methods of dealing with the pandemic through either marketisation, disaster capitalism or a strengthening of the state and some form of 'state capture'. Rather, alternatives around social movements and mutual aid are suggested drawing on anarchist and autonomist (anarchist/Marxist) perspectives. Although mutual aid is always subject to co-option by state authorities this book suggests new ways forward for resistance and the building of autonomous communities in the current pandemic crisis.

In theorising the relationship between COVID-19 and capitalism, class, crisis and resistance we draw on both Marxist and anarchist theory. In terms of Marxism, we use Marx (Marx 1976) as well as neo-Marxists such as Althusser in our arguments but we also draw on ideas from new work on 'value' (Postone 1980, 1993, 2017), value critique (Kurz 2012, 2014) and open Marxism (Bonefeld et al. 1992). We also use the work of cultural sociologists who draw on broader, more culturally orientated, manifestations of class war on the working class (namely Skeggs 2013). We do not consider the advent of COVID-19 as a significant 'break' from capitalism (the categories of value, labour and profit are still in operation) as capitalists remain fixated on the pursuit of profit and the expansion of its social universe of 'value' (Postone 1993) even as they require the state for bail-outs. Class relations and class struggle are inevitable relations in capitalist societies (Bonefeld et al. 1992) which are always antagonistic and cannot be finally mediated through social reform or the state. In terms of the latter, the state is not separate from capitalist relations (Postone 1993; Tenkle 2014) and cannot be repurposed for revolutionary purposes (Kurz 2012). In line with anarchist perspectives a vanguard approach to revolution is critiqued in favour of autonomous working-class struggle (Kurz 2012) with a sensitivity to the ways in which social policy (in this case pandemic policy) is used as a weapon against the working class (Skeggs 2013). Class war takes place on multiple levels and through cultural as well as economic means. Hence the work of sociologists who have specifically looked at the ways in which cultural manifestations of class power, and social policy, act as violence against the working class is used.

In the anarchist tradition the condition of resistance is the idea of the 'social principle' (an abstract theory), or 'mutual aid' (a correlate concrete practice). Anarchist theory, alongside autonomist Marxism, open Marxism and value theory, differs from theories that presume the state is essential. These theories posit the possibility of grassroots agency and the need to form non-capitalist autonomous lifeworlds to prefigure and build the conditions for resistance. In the anarchist tradition, a seminal text that we draw upon is Kropotkin's (1897) treatise on the historical rise of the state as a violent process of dispossession, enclosure and destruction of communal folk knowledge. The state aids the powerful interests of capitalists by seizing local institutions for the benefit of dominant minorities, imposing servitude before the law, and enforcing conformity of social roles within institutions (Ibid: 25). The individual is subjected and deprived of liberties, obliged to forget social ties based on free agreement and initiative in favour of a system where the state alone is able to create union between subjects. Kropotkin argues that revolutionaries who seek to achieve social change through state powers are misguided, because the essence of the state is to hinder the possibility of free society (Ibid: 10).

All conflicts and projects come to be arbitrated by the state, so one perspective is always repressed and silenced (Ibid: 33).

Kropotkin's alternative to the state is 'the social principle' which is the practice of free association, social solidarity and mutual aid, and he draws on a very wide range of case studies of human and animal groups to show that those who are strongest are those where individuals learn to co-operate and use mutual aid to support one another (Kropotkin 1902). The social principle is not idealised as conflict-free, but importantly conflicts can be debated and resolved without outside force, and problems large and small can generally be solved without unitarian co-ordinating authority (Kropotkin 1897). This idea was taken up by the British anarchist writer Colin Ward (1973), who we also draw upon in our understanding of society, who made the political argument that in much of everyday life groups like neighbourhood associations and musical subcultures are examples of anarchy in action, even if the groups stated aims are apolitical, from people with mainstream jobs and lives. Ward's approach to anarchism is tolerant and non-sectarian: the point is neither to pursue pure anarchism nor to build a one-off event, but rather, to build and expand the field of the social principle across as much of life as possible, until it gets to the point where it strains at the limits set by state and capital, and bursts out into the whole of society.

The idea of society as an authentic 'outside' to state and capitalist mediation and control in the form of a different social logic has been alluded to in different terminology by many different anarchist, anti-authoritarian, post-structuralist and non-statist Marxist philosophers, for example Negri's 'constituent power', Holloway's between 'power to' and 'power over' (Holloway 2005), Castoriadis' 'socially instituting imaginary' (Castoriadis 1998), Virno's (2004) multitude and exodus, Agamben's (1990) 'whatever-singularity' and Deleuze's concept (1983), drawing on Nietzsche, of 'active force'. Deep ecologists and eco-anarchists have extended the possibility of unalienated relationships beyond humans to the natural environment (e.g. Zerzan 2012: 23; Merchant 1980), and feminist and post-colonial thinkers have linked the domination of women and dispossession of indigenous people to the enclosure and destruction of local and folk knowledges, the reconstruction of which offers a potential site of resistance (Federici 2004; Mies 1986). There is also a political literature on horizontalism in Autonomous Social Movements (ASMs) of the late twentieth and early twenty-first centuries with an ethnographic element that places emphasis on movements that reconstruct direct/unmediated relationships, showing how these movements do not seek reformist change through statist structures, nor to seize state power, but rather to 'create free spaces in which self-determined decisions can be made autonomously and implemented directly' (Katsiaficas 1997: 5; see also Day 2005; Sitrin 2007; Graeber 2009). All of these ethnographic accounts echo Kropotkin's distinction between two different logics: a social logic of free association and direct, horizontal social relations defined in opposition to a hierarchical political logic which requires relationships to be mediated by a state, or emergent states such as a counter-hegemonic bloc or a fixed identity category. This distinction is an essential condition of possibility for anarchist theory, since the first premise of anarchism is that a stateless society is both possible and desirable, and the way to move towards it is by practicing it in the here-and-now rather than deferring to the future or relying on the leadership of vanguards.

While there are seemingly irreconcilable differences between most mainstream forms of Marxism and anarchist theory and practice, which have played out historically in fundamental splits in the Left, we do not believe that these splits are insurmountable when it comes to affinities between certain autonomous and open forms of Marxism, and the particular strains of socialist and communist anarchism we will also use. They share general libertarianism and critique of the state; anti-capitalism; sympathy for new social movements and tendency to broad-based (not just workplace) resistance, for example supporting ecology, anti-war, anti-nuclear, feminist, black movements; critique of alienation; valuing of active horizontal social life-force (commoning, social principle, affinity). They share central emphasis on critique of both state capture and capitalist commodification. Both valorise broadly horizontalist modes of struggle (rather than vanguardism) and similar visions of revolution as arising from prefiguration and direct action and proliferation of everyday connections and grassroots struggles.

There are also some important differences, which might lead to occasional productive tensions between the two authors of this book, but we believe nothing fundamentally contradictory. These include differences in focus on source material and terminology. Open Marxists make heavy use of Marx when referring to certain Marxian categories, even if used in nonstandard ways (e.g. capital, totality, class/value-struggle, fetishism), whereas anarchists tend to rely on canonical anarchist texts, and therefore rely on anarchist terminology (e.g. totalising or hierarchical relations, social/political principle, non-hierarchy, dis-alienation). Open Marxists mostly view the state as a terrain of struggle and a subordinate effect of class relations, anarchists see it as a primary antagonist. The open Marxist pole of our perspective has a more explicit tendency towards human mass collectivism, that the creative life-force exists at a collective level of human labour, and individual-level phenomena are alienated (which might restrict which struggles they can embrace and how). Some forms of anarchism are happier with small-group actions and subcultural isolation or self-isolation than open Marxists are; and the more anarchist pole in our argument is more focused on local community action than national policy context or population response. By the same token, the open/neo-Marxist pole is sometimes happier with some forms of conventional politics, working within institutions and using formal organisations strategically—whilst resisting and acting against and beyond. Views of 'the subject' are slightly different; with Marxists viewing the subject as socially constituted, with anarchists agreeing but viewing a kernel of authentic desires (which form the basis of within-system autonomous resistance). However, these differences are rather subtle, and they ought not to detract from the force of the argument, in fact the structure of this book plays on the particular strengths of the different theories, with Chap. 3 using variations on Marxist theory to critique the current policy context and to expose the unequal capitalist relations it supports, and Chap. 4 using anarchist theories to understand the perspective of autonomous social movements mobilising mutual aid.

Obviously, this book represents a 'live sociology' of a crisis at one point in time—at what might be called the 'foothills' of the pandemic. This analysis tracked the 'first wave' of the pandemic through the initial idea of quarantine, to the lockdown 'stay home' phase until the changing of messaging and emphasis to 'stay alert'. All sociology dates but there is considerable risk in writing a book on this topic when the pandemic might escalate further so as to make writing on this topic at this stage seem trivial, or (in an extremely unlikely scenario) the virus may mutate to a less harmful strain or a miracle vaccine may be discovered. However, the principles of the work remain applicable to other pandemics and crises of this type as well as to the ways in which the state and capital attempt to colonise mutual aid and social movements in a crisis. In terms of sources, this book was written based on information from government directives, press articles and news reports that were in the public domain. No human subjects were involved in the research and this book makes no use of personal information. It was produced during the first wave of the coronavirus pandemic in the UK March–May 2020. The authors have no conflicts of interests in the writing of this book.

Throughout this book we will refer to the disease as COVID-19 but also refer as 'coronavirus' and the 'virus'. We hope that readers, particularly from the sciences, will be tolerant of the flexibility of our terminology.

References

Agamben, G. (1990). *The Coming Community*. Minneapolis: University of Minnesota Press.

Bonefeld, W., Gunn, R., & Psychopedis, K. (1992). *Open Marxism*. London: Pluto Press.

Castoriadis, C. (1998). *The Imaginary Institution of Society*. Cambridge, MA: MIT Press.

Day, R. J. F. (2005). *Gramsci Is Dead: Anarchist Currents in the Newest Social Movements*. London: Pluto.

Deleuze, G. (1983). *Nietzsche and Philosophy*. London: Bloomsbury.

Federici, S. (2004). *Caliban and the Witch: Women, the Body and Primitive Accumulation*. New York: Autonomedia.

Graeber, D. (2009). *Direct Action: An Ethnography*. Oakland: AK Press.

Harvey, D. (2000). *The Condition of Postmodernity*. Cambridge, MA: Blackwell.

Holloway, J. (2005). *Change the World Without Taking Power*. London: Pluto.

Katsiaficas, G. (1997 [2006]). *The Subversion of Politics: European Autonomous Social Movements and the Decolonization of Everyday Life*. Oakland: AK Press.

Kropotkin, P. (1897). *The State: Its Historic Role* (V. Richards, Trans. 1997). London: Freedom Press.

Kropotkin, P. (1902). *Mutual Aid: A Factor of Evolution*, ed. W. Jonson (2014). CreateSpace Independent Publishing Platform.

Kurz, R. (2012). *No Revolution Anywhere: The Life and Death of Capitalism*. London: Chronos Publications.

Kurz, R. (2014). The Crisis of Exchange Value: Science as a Productive Force, Productive Labour and Capitalist Reproduction. In N. Larsen, M. Nilges, J. Robinson, & N. Brown (Eds.), *Marxism and the Critique of Value* (pp. 17–76). Chicago: MCM' Publishing.

Marx, K. (1976). *Capital: A Critique of Political Economy, Volume 1*. London: Penguin.

Marx, K., & Engels, F. (2002). *The Communist Manifesto*. London: Penguin.

Merchant, C. (1980). *The Death of Nature: Women, Ecology and the Scientific Revolution*. New York: Harper Collins.

Mies, M. (1986 [2014]). *Patriarchy and Accumulation on a World Scale: Women in the International Division of Labour*. London: Zed Books.

Postone, M. (1980). Anti-Semitism and National Socialism: Notes on the German Reaction to "Holocaust". *New German Critique, 19*, 97–115. https://doi.org/10.2307/487974.

Postone, M. (1993). *Time, Labor and Social Domination*. Cambridge: Cambridge University Press.

Postone, M. (2017). The Current Crisis and the Anachronism of Value: A Marxian Reading. *Continental Thought and Theory: A Journal of Intellectual Freedom, 1*(4), 38–54.

Sitrin, M. (2007). *Horizontalism: Voices of Popular Power in Argentina*. Edinburgh: AK Press.

Skeggs, B. (2013). *Class, Self, Culture*. London: Routledge.

Tenkle, N. (2014). Value and Crisis: Basic Questions. In N. Larsen, M. Nilges, J. Robinson, & N. Brown (Eds.), *Marxism and the Critique of Value* (pp. 1–16). Chicago: MCM' Publishing.

Virno, P. (2004). *A Grammar of the Multitude*. Cambridge, MA: MIT Press.

Ward, C. (1973). *Anarchy in Action*. London: Aldgate Press.

Zerzan, J. (2012). *Future Primitive Revisited*. Port Townsend: Feral House.

2

The *Viracene* and Capitalism

John Preston and Rhiannon Firth

Introduction: COVID-19 and the Abstractions of Capital

It could be argued that the term *viracene* should be used to refer to the current process of viral pandemic destruction but unlike the *Anthropocene* this is a short-term crust on a wider planetary devastation and asset stripping of nature. Any phase that can be constructed is ephemeral when compared to the devastation of *capitalism* which sees itself as being eternal, operating on scales from the viral to the cosmic and unavoidably destructive of humanity and nature. Both Marxist and anarchist analyses of capitalism contend that, whether in pandemic or not, capitalism is always in crisis. For Marxists, crisis emerges from the conditions of capitalist commodity production which necessitates the antagonistic relationship between labour and capital (Bonefeld et al. 1992) whereby the substance of value in capitalism (labour power) consistently undermines its own ability to produce value (Kurz 2012, 2014) as capitalists are compelled (by the profit motive) to replace labour with physical capital (Marx 1976; Postone 1993, 2017). For anarchists, this crisis is exacerbated by the imposition of hierarchical control and ordering over national territories by the nation state which alienates

© The Author(s) 2020

J. Preston, R. Firth, *Coronavirus, Class and Mutual Aid in the United Kingdom,*
https://doi.org/10.1007/978-3-030-57714-8_2

and fragments social and community relations to the extent that it renders people incapable of contributing to decisions that affect their health directly, and of helping each other through mutual aid (Kropotkin 1897, 1902; Ward 1973).

With this background, COVID-19, the *viracene*, appears within a 2020 context whereby the world economy was already in danger of crisis with a massive backlash against the very capitalist idea of a 'world market'. Trade wars between China and the United States, rising economic nationalism and isolation (the UK Brexit vote being one example of this) and declining profits in various economic sectors (including airplane and automotive production) had produced concerns about what the next area of capitalist profitability was going to be. Industry 4.0, the idea that industry could benefit from the principle of platform capitalism, artificial intelligence (AI) and technological solutions that have revolutionised the services sector were contenders for this. Another was the 'green industrial revolution', supported by hedge funds and technology entrepreneurs, which had the advantage of significant public support and a quasi-revolutionary, but often reactionary (in terms of its comfort with capitalist business models), fervour (Bernes 2019). Yet another was the idea of 'smart cities' using sensors placed throughout the urban environment to collect data and use it to automate infrastructure, resource and service management (Ruhlandt 2018).

In this context of capitalist crisis as an eternal event in capitalism, albeit with temporal and situational (historical) features, it is difficult to see whether COVID-19 was a cause of a visible economic crisis or as a welcome relief for capitalists and states to restate what was already happening in a capitalist world economy. During February, stock markets fell by an equivalent which was not seen since the 2008 financial crisis and commodity prices became increasingly erratic. There were cuts to (already historically low) interest rates. On supermarket shelves around the world and in online shops supplies of masks of various kinds, painkillers, toilet rolls, hand-sanitisers, dried and canned foods and soap disappeared. Where there were supplies prices were increased and price-gouging became common as retailers also increased their prices. There was a sudden realisation by employers, who had previously been obsessed with replacing workers with AI and robots, that workers would not be able or willing to work. In context of pandemic crisis, employers realised that they really needed workers and employees realised that they could not necessarily depend on a long-term replacement income from the state if they had to self-isolate for an extended period of time. In the UK the state stepped in to *temporarily* pay a proportion of worker's wages under the furlough scheme. Despite efforts by WHO (World Health Organisation) and other countries to distinguish the origin of the virus from a particular national context (previous epidemics had been named 'Asian flu' or 'Spanish flu') there was an increase in xenophobia and racism. For some organisations this resulted in massive contradictions. European universities, for example, who depended on Chinese students, realised that these students would possibly not be able to travel to study. This resulted in a rush towards offering online courses which would not necessarily appeal to such students. Circuits of production, consumption and distribution were disrupted or simply halted.

In the current COVID-19 crisis the whole economic system appears to be 'contaminated' from banknotes to packaging and supply chains. Labour itself becomes a possible source of viral contamination. Fears that COVID-19 can spread via money and commodities were particularly salient in terms of the objectification of capitalist relations. We already experience 'things' in capitalism in a fetishised state (Marx 1976; Tenkle 2014). Commodities appear to be things of use (use value) and of exchange (exchange value) but are in reality reified forms of human labour. Money is also a commodity (for exchange) which is the ultimate objectified form of value. Objectively, these things are human constructs which (in any case) comprised human essences (labour power). Money may be already literally contaminated with human sweat, urine and faeces and the whiff of consumed cocaine but it is also *embodied flesh* in terms of the labour power that produced the commodities which were sold for money at a value greater than the money that was applied in their production (Marx 1976). Similarly, there were fears around packaging as if it were the only human component of a commodity whereas the *commodity itself* is made by human labour. Pandemics awaken us to the sociality of commodity production in all of its forms and the ridiculousness of the asocial nature of market relations in capitalism. We realise that we are part of society and that we are also vulnerable to the relations of others. We indulge in what has been called 'panic buying' by hoarding certain commodities (particularly hand sanitiser, toilet rolls and pasta in this current pandemic) whilst rejecting others (such as holidays and air travel). Butler (2004) considers our sociality in terms of how far others can be the 'undoing' of us and how relations between ourselves and the boundaries between ourselves and others are permeable but relations of class allow some (the ruling class) to escape labour and tactile consumption. In a Marxist analysis what is seemingly concrete obscures and inverts the real social relations. Analogously, Postone (1980) considers the Nazi Holocaust by analysing how Nazi propaganda concretised the nature of 'Aryan' German labour whilst making the labour and investments of Jewish people seemingly abstract and dishonest. COVID-19 presents an equally false dichotomy between the abstract nature of money and commodities which are asocial and their contaminating properties as concrete items. People become increasingly concerned with increasing the consumption of what appear to be insubstantial commodities such as 'contactless' payment and 'streaming' services which enter the house or mobile phone wirelessly. COVID-19 is a perfect pandemic for an economic reality of the immaterial so as not to 'connect' with the reality of physical money, commodities or others who might harbour the virus. The COVID-19 pandemic reminds us of the visceral nature of capitalism. The precarity of working lives becomes central as those of us who are working class, without inherited wealth or savings, realise that we are living paycheque to paycheque. Despite the ways in which capitalism attempts to interpolate life as frictionless with contactless payments and unlimited home delivery of a cornucopia of commodities COVID-19 brings us face to face with the reality of commodity production and demand and supply. In particular, working-class bodies, and working-class jobs, in areas such as construction and food delivery, become increasingly pathologised as visceral, physical, labour is thought to be a source of 'contamination'.

Class and Class War as Multi-Dimensional

Capitalism creates its own dimensionality. The essence of capital, as self-valorising value (Postone 1993) in the abstract is not tied to concrete ideas of space and time and consistently seeks to destroy and disestablish those laws (Harvey 2000). This might seem esoteric and even occult. On the one hand capitalism seems to operate by the rules of classical political economy and classical physics. An orthodox political economy approach might envisage workers as selling their labour time to a capitalist who produces products which are sold for money yielding a profit, the money is then reinvested by the capitalist. This happens in 'real time' in that it involves concrete production, circulation and exchange (realisation). In a Marxist analysis capitalism consistently aims to increase exploitation and economise time and space to maintain profits. Every moment of labour time, and less than moments if possible, must be maximised. Circulation and valorisation should take place as quickly as possible, preferably instantaneously, and most preferably before even the commodity is produced (Postone 1993). Constantly undermining its own basis, capitalists invest in technology and creating new commodities and new markets at every scale (Marx and Engels 2002). Hence capitalism creates new dimensions of commodities, markets and time (what Postone (1993) refers to as abstract time).

This has two implications. Firstly, that capitalism itself operates at every level of dimensionality and a level of abstract dimensionality which is the 'real' nature of capitalism itself. Capitalism is both sub-quantum and universal macroscopic in reach. No physical entity of any scale is beyond marketisation (although anarchists would argue that where there is intentionality at the level of *desire* communities can become autonomous unless or until they are repressed or co-opted). Secondly, that COVID-19, as an entity that exists in a capitalist reality, enables the creation of a multiplicity of new markets and commodity forms, not only in the form of a cure, but also in terms of markets in preparedness and protection, devouring and reconstituting forms of labour in health, care, protection and policing and creating increased financialisation in futures and other financial assets. As well as in markets in viral treatments it is technically possible to gain a form of property right over a virus. For example, in 2012 Erasmus Medical Centre patented the genetic sequence of MERS-CoV. There are questions in terms of the extent to which a virus can be patented without modification, and it may not be possible in certain geographical territories, but there are already discussions concerning the possibility of patenting elements of SARS-CoV-2. This would be in terms of aspects of the sequencing of this particular coronavirus genome.

Like any form of property, capitalists attempt to accumulate by dispossession (Harvey 2000) by securing a natural form, namely the possession of properties of the virus, as intellectual property and its exploitation for future rents and profits. COVID-19, in opening up new markets and forms of commodity, produces the potential for capitalism to expand its 'social universe' of commodities in all directions (Rikowski 2000) but this also produces new fields and arenas for class conflict. COVID-19 will bring new forms of scientific labour into the enterprise of vaccine and (potentially) virus production hence a commodity is being produced on a viral engineering scale with all of the multi-dimensional aspects of class conflict that exist for other commodities. The viral and anti-viral industries present a new opportunity for profit and one would expect finance capital to move from less profitable areas of the economy to the 'COVID-19' industry. The mobility and spontaneity of capital and its flows are (as remarked on in the Communist Manifesto, Marx and Engels 2002) a remarkable modernist achievement but also alert us that the motion of capital is continuous as it is always in crisis and always in conflict with the living force of labour (Rikowski 2000). Although capitalism consistently seeks new markets and opportunities for exploitation, we would reject the metaphor of a 'virus' for capitalism itself and it is not the one which is appropriate here. Rather, capitalism operates on a multitude of scales and creates its own scalar nature in terms of the alien dimension of value. Capital moves between social forms, not in a viral sense, but in a way that it is inimical to life itself. It is in that sense only that it functions in a way similar to a killer pandemic, in opposition to living labour. In the UK, as the 'stay home' message moves to 'stay alert' on 10th May workers are urged to return to work across various sectors to maintain capitalist production and circulation. In doing so they risk their personal safety and health, and that of their families. The 'sacrifice' of living labour into dead labour is one which is, in any case, demanded every day by capitalism. In working-class lives disease, illness and early death are familiar consequences of class war (and in opposition to this there are gallows humour, resistance and solidarity) but these are accelerated through working in a pandemic.

Viruses As 'Forces of Nature'

Even if COVID-19 cannot always be fully commodified it acts as what might be called a 'force of nature' within capitalist society (Marx 1976). 'Forces of nature' are those forces, which might be natural, or of human origin, which facilitate the functioning of capital in some sense. There are several examples of this in Marx's work including natural forces such as tides, rain and the sun, which can act to speed the manufacture and transportation of goods or the production of crops and forces of human origin such as roads and communications infrastructures that can reduce circulation times and increase the chance that capital investment is valorised in the sale of products. A virus is a tool of capitalist mobilisation in that it is a 'natural force' that propels certain forms of capital. For example, it destroys certain branches of industry and leads to new branches of industry in developing research tools and vaccines and other civilian and military operations. COVID-19 is becoming part of capital itself in terms of being inextricably linked to these processes now and in the foreseeable future. This idea of a 'force of nature' separate from capitalism can also produce an analysis by governments of the virus arising from outside of capitalism and as a threat to capitalism. The virus appears to be an external entity threatening commodity production, circulation and exchange. Capital (as involving self-valorising value) cannot survive without these processes. Hence the state can justify 'extraordinary measures' to save capitalism and the notion of worker sacrifice in terms of returning to work. In the UK there has been an emphasis on loans and other financial packages to business of an extraordinary level and the changing of laws and regulations to make capital more flexible. For example, restrictions on pubs and restaurants being able to deliver takeaway food have been lifted and safety requirements regarding Personal Protective Equipment (PPE) for care homes and the NHS (National Health Service) have been relaxed. The state acts as a form of finance capital but without changing the centrality of capitalism as a system of value production. This is a transfer of risk from capitalists to the government. In other countries, such as Greece, perhaps because of previous austerity which has favoured a strong state, the approach has focussed more on the national takeover of private resources and an authoritarian approach but in all Western countries the nexus between capital, state and authoritarian governance is equally strong and even welcomed (albeit temporarily) by large proportions of the population.

Eugenics, Surplus Population and 'Viral Immiseration'

Capitalism is contradictory as it needs labour to survive whilst consistently expelling labour as it replaces workers with fixed capital. Even before COVID-19 capitalists expressed concerns regarding a 'residual' population whose jobs would be replaced through technology and new organisational forms. The substitution of labour by AI, robotics and machine learning, without new industries to develop jobs, was a common trope in news media worldwide. A significant part of the move towards restrictions on immigration and an increasingly populist and authoritarian agenda was that immigrants could be replaced through technology. Rather than 'native' workers, robots and AI would take over the role of immigrant labour.

The problem of 'excess' labour and technological unemployment is not new to capitalism. Marx's use of 'surplus' population cuts through several of his concepts. In many ways, the human host of the unique commodity 'labour power' is tolerated by capitalists and life itself is an inconvenience to capital as well as being an entity that must be tamed if the capitalist is going to maximise the rate of exploitation. The costs of sickness and fatigue are frequently passed from the capitalist to the worker or to the state form where possible. Surplus population also refers to the 'industrial reserve army' of the unemployed, the size of which increases and decreases according to the demand for labour power in various industries (Marx 1976). It can also refer to those portions of the proletariat whose labour is not utilised in various industries due to legal or moral restrictions on the basis of some characteristic (such as age). These various forms of 'surplus population' are often the subject of discussions on eugenics that have re-emerged recently in work on evolutionary biology and psychology, IQ testing and socio-genomics on the right. However, discourses of over-population on the grounds of environmentalism have also emerged on the left.

This is reflected in various ways in the current COVID-19 crisis. Some politicians have a belief that the virus should be allowed to reap its way through the population. On the 'Good Morning Britain' television programme on 9th March 2020, Boris Johnson stated that 'One of the theories is perhaps you could *take it on the chin*, take it all in one go and allow Coronavirus to move through the population without really taking as many draconian measures'. This rhetoric of a robust population needing to 'get things done' has obvious parallels with the Brexit slogan adopted by Johnson: 'Get Brexit Done'. The reporting of the age distribution of COVID-19 victims shows that older populations (particularly those over 70) are particularly susceptible to the virus. Some forms of reporting in the media have suggested that this means that COVID-19 is not particularly serious when compared to other infections such as pandemic flu. Underlying these assumptions is a particularly capitalist view of the diminished value of human life of those who are older than 70 since they are not often active in the labour market. In addition, the way in which a xenophobic portrayal of the virus as affecting people of a particular nationality such as Chinese people is used negatively in the popular press and on social media. This has resulted in a number of xenophobic and racist attacks on Chinese people in the UK. Thirdly, arguments concerning healthy practices and unhealthy areas (e.g. that things will 'improve' when the temperature increases and the virus moves to the Southern Hemisphere) are elements of eugenic thought that enter into media and social media conversations. All of these elements are part of a capitalist ideology of the value (or not) of certain populations.

In these circumstances, concerns of social justice are particularly obscured and the lack of attention to these issues has been previously remarked on by other authors in their analysis of pandemic preparedness. Some of these issues were foreseen in terms of a future pandemic influenza epidemic, which could be particularly applied to the coronavirus:

> In preparing to deal with the likely challenges of an influenza pandemic, including very limited future vaccine supply and lack of availability of appropriate antiviral medications, all levels of governmental public health should focus on inherent barriers to a fair distribution of benefits and burdens. These include entrenched racial, ethnic, and socioeconomic disparities in health outcomes, lack of bidirectional communication, and unequal access to medical care, as well as the conditions that make these populations vulnerable in the first place. Even during winters with influenza from flu strains that have changed only a bit, low vaccination coverage among ethnic and racial minorities and persons living in and near poverty is a persistent problem, particularly for hard-to-reach populations (eg, injection drug users, elderly shut-ins, and undocumented immigrants). Failure to prepare to respond appropriately to the needs of these populations during an emergency can serve to exacerbate racial, ethnic, and socioeconomic disparities in infectious disease outcomes, and thus may leave even those in the dominant population in a more vulnerable position. (Kayman and Ablorh-Odjidja 2006)

Garoon and Duggan (2008) in a critical discourse analysis of thirty-seven pandemic preparedness plans reveal the way in which the disadvantaged are 'masked and neglected'. None of the plans explicitly referenced groups who were economically disadvantaged. They suggest that:

> Failure to address social as well as biological vulnerability thereby poses the danger of repeating the differential trends in mortality observed in 1918— meaning individuals and groups disadvantaged in the *status quo ante* would suffer a significantly disproportionate force of mortality. Thus, the plans' apparently uncontroversial aim of minimizing morbidity and mortality should in fact raise critical questions: *Whose* illness? *Whose* deaths? (Garoon and Duggan 2008, 1135–1136)

As can be seen, the realm of eugenic policy for pandemics applies to the classed and socially unjust aspects of the ways in which populations are expected to be managed. Indeed, it is quite possible that once state support for workers is cut back, there is a return to austerity and capitalists depend on a process of 'viral immiseration' (forcing workers back to work even if they become ill or die from the virus) by reducing wage supports and benefits to 'starve' workers back to dangerous work.

Although the emphasis of this book is primarily on class and hierarchy, it must be noted that the biopolitical and necropolitical consequences of the pandemic also apply unequally to people according to structural inequalities associated with other intersecting characteristics such as race, gender, ability/disability, age and sexuality. As has been discussed, the racial and ethnic dimensions of COVID-19 have been emphasised by some populist politicians, for example, Donald Trump has referred to the virus as the 'Chinese Virus' reflecting fears in the administration of Chinese domination of trade and a long-standing anti-Asian and nativist streak in US politics. This is played out at the micro level in terms of micro-aggressions against Asian people for wearing masks, travelling on public transport and even physical aggression in some cases. There has also been a xenophobic backlash on social media against small (primarily Asian-run) shops in the UK that are selling products such as toilet rolls and hand sanitiser at high prices. There are also racialised implications for already disproportionately immiserated communities, particularly (in the US and UK) the working-class black community, whose lack of access to good food, housing and community and safety renders them much more vulnerable to not only the biological dangers of the virus but also to physically and mentally unsafe conditions during lockdown, and disproportionately repressive security and policing measures if they inadvertently break rules that were made without consideration for their conditions. There are also gendered aspects of the pandemic in terms of assumptions of who will provide 'care' when state resources, such as schooling, are withdrawn alongside a middle-class emphasis on household management and home education, as will be considered in the next chapter.

As the virus has a differential impact on those with certain underlying conditions and older individuals most governments have provided special protection for those groups. In the UK as of the end of March 2020 plans were put into practice to 'shield' 1.5 million people from the virus by advising them to stay at home for twelve weeks with the possibility of food parcel delivery to their homes. This involves the state making value judgements and this approach has also been criticised in the UK as being part of a 'herd immunity' approach of reducing social distancing so that economic activity can accelerate. This policy has also been advocated by the President of the United States. The 'sacrifice' of some individuals for the 'greater good' of the economy has obvious eugenic implications. Finally, sexuality is indirectly invoked as the HIV epidemic (where gay men were amongst the original group of victims and which has, homophobically, been linked since with this group) has been cited by a British politician from the Brexit Party, Anne Widdicombe:

> I'm all for sensible precautions but I cannot help feeling that we are going mad over coronavirus. We have had the scare of SARS, bird flu, Ebola and of course AIDS. None proved as devastating as feared. We need a sense of proportion in the face of the financial markets going into meltdown, aeroplanes being grounded and shops shutting their doors. It is nasty but, given the recovery rate, it is not the Black Death. (The Independent 2020)

To consider HIV/AIDS as a 'scare' is to make assumptions about victimhood centred on heteronormative, and anti-scientific, standpoints of the virus as only impacting on certain populations. There are numerous ways in which these intersectional characteristics operate with the classed dimensions of oppression and these will be referred to throughout this book.

Commodification, Disaster Capitalism and the Repressive State Apparatus

As considered above, at the time of writing capitalism has already produced a range of new commodities in response to COVID-19 directly related to health and vaccines but it also produces commodities that are part of 'prepping' for disasters. Prepping has, until recently, been seen to be an activity which was on the fringe of societies, indulged in by conspiracy theorists who often have right wing, or otherwise extremist, views. The ruling class, who have been buying islands, bunkers and private security militias, have made prepping respectable and there are now a whole range of elite commodity lines for the upper middle classes including high-quality masks:

> "En route to Paris," Gwyneth Paltrow wrote on Instagram last week, beneath a shot of herself on an airplane heading to Paris Fashion Week and wearing a black face mask. "I've already been in this movie," she added, referring to her role in the 2011 disease thriller "Contagion." "Stay safe." Ms. Paltrow did not pose with just any mask, unlike, say, Kate Hudson and Bella Hadid, who also recently posted selfies wearing cheaper, disposable masks. The Goop founder and influencer of influencers instead opted for a sleek "urban air mask" by a Swedish company, Airinum, which features five layers of filtration and an "ultrasmooth and skin-friendly finish." (Williams and Bromwich 2020)

For the ruling class the virus has displaced environmental crisis, nuclear war and existential threats of AI as the most prescient crisis. As one of the authors has discussed previously (Preston 2019) it is the ruling class, rather than survivalist blue-collar Americans, who are the primary market for prepping in contemporary crises. It has been reported that the ruling class are retreating to private islands and bunkers, paying for their own private tests and treatments and advancing doctors and physicians huge sums of money to accompany them to their retreats. This allows the ruling class to resist the barriers to travel that have been imposed on other citizens through the chartering of private flights:

Adam Twidell, chief executive of the private jet booking service PrivateFly, said his firm was continuing to see a jump in bookings as wealthy people arranged evacuation flights home from high-risk countries. He said: "Many are from groups which include elderly passengers or those with health conditions that make them particularly concerned about exposure to crowds on airline flights. We've just flown a group back to London from the south of France, with an immunocompromised passenger on board". Twidell said other rich clients were arranging flights out of the UK and other European countries in advance of the possible introduction of nationwide quarantine measures following Italy's lead. (Neate 2020)

The COVID-19 pandemic occurs at a particularly *good* time for capitalism in terms of the ways in which the permanent crisis of capitalism is realised in the economic domain. A number of factors have led to a recent world economic downturn including the increase in tariff and trade barriers and the fall in profitability in manufacturing and service industries. COVID-19 has been associated with a fall in the stock, commodities and futures markets in a number of countries and a decline in the shares of companies associated with aviation and travel. In terms of the current ways in which consumer capitalism is constituted the virus occurs at a time when there is a plethora of social media, streaming and home delivery services available. The ubiquity of the smartphone and smart devices in the home means that individuals can be personally entertained and satisfied in quarantine and isolation. As long as people have access to electricity, wi-fi and/or wireless technologies (including the new technology of 5G) they can gain access to social media and a wealth of entertainment. Streaming services such as Netflix and the recently launched Disney+ (the timing of the latter is exceptionally fortunate) alongside gaming technologies means that some middle-class individuals do not have to step outside to work, play and interact with others. Home delivery services mean that fortunate individuals do not have to go outside to gain access to food and supplies. Platforms such as Zoom and Skype allow people to attend meetings from their own homes. This produces a new type of (middle-class) consumer and worker, the *uncontaminated*, who have a seemingly frictionless and independent existence separate from the visceral nature of capitalism in terms of touching commodities outside of the home in shops or producing them in the workplace. This is, of course, illusionary in that the asocial nature of this existence involves multiple interactions with commodity production involving living labour. All of this seemingly frictionless and virtual activity is a direct product of the labour of the exploited working class who are working in pandemic conditions.

The crisis creates a number of new market sectors and allows for what Klein (2008) has called 'disaster capitalism' or the ways in which capitalism engineers and uses 'forces of nature' to profit from disaster, war and accident. In the case of COVID-19 the disaster allows for a new specification of state priorities for health and social care. Where there have been COVID-19 outbreaks there has been an increased demand for beds and treatments, particularly in intensive care units (ITUs) so that demand rapidly exceeds supply. In the care sector, sickness amongst carers and nurses has led to a situation where people, particularly older citizens or those with complex health needs, forgo care. These situations present an opportunity for 'disaster capitalism' involving expansion of the private sector into what was formerly state provision so that private hospitals, and associated facilities, can address the care needs of patients. It increases the demand for technical solutions in care such as the use of 'Alexa' type devices to provide contact with the elderly and sick. In education, if teachers and lecturers are sick or absent (or campuses are shut), technological solutions such as distance learning can be employed to provide teaching and learning where staff and students are unable to attend classes. What was previously provided by the state can now be offered by the market and COVID-19 provides the opportunity, and excuse, for the private sector to enter what were previously markets that were limited by state provision. In this way capital can expand into new markets in the search for increased profits.

Capital can also use the pandemic to establish new modes of production, or to intensify existing tendencies. The importance of logistics for home delivery, for example, has become extremely important in the current pandemic and will tend to increase the move to the 'Amazonification' of capitalism. In parallel, for financial sectors, COVID-19 modifies existing financial products and allows for the development of new financial mechanisms. In the case of insurance, insurers quickly modified contracts and introduced new products for travel and trade to account for the spread of the virus. This allowed insurers to potentially gain increased profits from new markets. Similarly, futures markets are extended to produce new forms of financial product for pandemics.

Whilst some areas of the world market contract the crisis allows for the extension of the state in the service of capital. Part of the criticism that Western countries made of China's reaction to the pandemic was the use of surveillance technologies and enforced quarantine in the COVID-19 outbreak. However, capitalist countries (and China could be classed as a 'state capitalist' country) also have their own mechanisms for containing the virus. Althusser (2001) refers to the 'Repressive State Apparatus' as the set of institutions and bodies that can enforce certain ruling class priorities in a crisis. In the case of COVID-19 the police and the army have been introduced as a major aspect of the management of the crisis in various countries. In the UK the police have been asked to enforce the rules concerning people staying at home and the movement of people with the ability to impose fines and prison sentences and the army are increasingly involved in logistics and setting up hospitals. Ultimately, the ending of the 'furlough' or 'job retention' scheme and mass unemployment are used as a form of 'viral immiseration' so that workers need to return or face the end of state support.

Conclusion

This chapter has advanced the argument that the COVID-19 pandemic has a direct relationship with capitalism and class which is not always disadvantageous for capital. Capitalism is a multi-dimensional and dynamic form of social mediation that operates at all levels, including the viral, and even the RNA code of the virus itself can be commodified. Viruses are mobilised by capital as a 'force of nature' that can then be used to increase profits. Excess populations can be exterminated 'naturally' through viral or xenophobic means in ways that benefit capital. Disaster capitalism extends the boundaries of both the market and state enforcement. Capitalism is not sympathetic to any form of life that it cannot commodify, accepts those begrudgingly, and that includes coronaviruses as well as worker's bodies. However, capital adapts and it is necessary for the survival of capitalism to expand into new markets and make profits where class is reproduced and classed bodies are marked through state and capitalist practices and processes. We now move to consider those classed elements of preparing for the COVID-19 epidemic in the UK in terms of behavioural science, panic-buying, altruism and quarantine.

References

Althusser, L. (2001). *Lenin and Philosophy*. New York: Monthly Review Press.

Bernes, J. (2019, Spring). Between the Devil and the Green New Deal. *Commune Mag*, Issue 2. https://communemag.com/between-the-devil-and-the-green-new-deal/. Accessed 25 May 2020.

Bonefeld, W., Gunn, R., & Psychopedis, K. (1992). *Open Marxism*. London: Pluto Press.

Butler, J. (2004). *Precarious Life: The Power of Mourning and Violence*. London: Verso.

Garoon, J., & Duggan, P. (2008). Discourses of Disease, Discourses of Disadvantage: A Critical Analysis of National Pandemic Influenza Preparedness Plans. *Social Science & Medicine, 67*(7), 1133–1142. https://doi.org/10.1016/j.socscimed.2008.06.020.

Harvey, D. (2000). *The Condition of Postmodernity*. Cambridge, MA: Blackwell.

Kayman, H., & Ablorh-Odjidja, A. (2006). Revisiting Public Health Preparedness. *Journal of Public Health Management and Practice, 12*(4), 373–380. https://doi.org/10.1097/00124784-200607000-00011.

Klein, N. (2008). *The Shock Doctrine*. London: Penguin.

Kropotkin, P. (1897). *The State: Its Historic Role* (V. Richards, Trans. 1997). London: Freedom Press.

Kropotkin, P. (1902). *Mutual Aid: A Factor of Evolution*, ed. W. Jonson (2014). CreateSpace Independent Publishing Platform.

Kurz, R. (2012). *No Revolution Anywhere: The Life and Death of Capitalism*. London: Chronos Publications.

Kurz, R. (2014). The Crisis of Exchange Value: Science as a Productive Force, Productive Labour and Capitalist Reproduction. In N. Larsen, M. Nilges, J. Robinson, & N. Brown (Eds.), *Marxism and the Critique of Value* (pp. 17–76). Chicago: MCM' Publishing.

Marx, K. (1976). *Capital: A Critique of Political Economy, Volume 1.* London: Penguin.

Marx, K., & Engels, F. (2002). *The Communist Manifesto.* London: Penguin.

Neate, R. (2020, May 21). *Super-Rich Jet Off to Disaster Bunkers Amid Coronavirus Outbreak.* Retrieved from: https://www.theguardian.com/world/2020/mar/11/disease-dodging-worried-wealthy-jet-off-to-disaster-bunkers

Postone, M. (1980). Anti-Semitism and National Socialism: Notes on the German Reaction to "Holocaust". *New German Critique, 19,* 97. https://doi.org/10.2307/487974.

Postone, M. (1993). *Time, Labor and Social Domination.* Cambridge: Cambridge University Press.

Postone, M. (2017). The Current Crisis and the Anachronism of Value: A Marxian Reading. *Continental Thought and Theory: A Journal of Intellectual Freedom, 1*(4), 38–54.

Preston, J. (2019). *Grenfell Tower: Preparedness, Race and Disaster Capitalism.* London: Palgrave. 3319968513. 978-3-319-96850-6.

Rikowski, G. (2000, September 7–10). *Messing with the Explosive Commodity: School Improvement, Educational Research and Labour-Power in the Era of Global Capitalism.* Paper presented at the British Educational Research Association Conference, Cardiff University.

Ruhlandt, R. W. S. (2018). The Governance of Smart Cities: A Systematic Literature Review. *Cities, 81,* 1–23.

Tenkle, N. (2014). Value and Crisis: Basic Questions. In N. Larsen, M. Nilges, J. Robinson, & N. Brown (Eds.), *Marxism and the Critique of Value* (pp. 1–16). Chicago: MCM' Publishing.

The Independent. (2020, May 21). *Ann Widdecombe Criticised After Saying Coronavirus Will Not Be 'As Devastating as Feared' by 'Comparing' It to the AIDS Epidemic.* Retrieved from: https://www.indy100.com/article/ann-widdecombe-coronavirus-aids-hiv-epidemic-twitter-response-9402006

Ward, C. (1973). *Anarchy in Action.* London: Aldgate Press.

Williams, A., & Bromwich, J. (2020, May 21) *The Rich Are Preparing for Coronavirus Differently.* Retrieved from: https://www.nytimes.com/2020/03/05/style/the-rich-are-preparing-for-coronavirus-differently.html

3

Classed Practices: Pandemic Preparedness in the UK

John Preston

A Global Pandemic

The World Health Organisation (WHO) have recently classified COVID-19 as a global pandemic. This is largely a matter of terminology, but a global pandemic means that the disease has crossed many national boundaries and exponentially infected a large number of people. Like all disasters, pandemics expose marked differences between health systems and exacerbate existing social inequalities. In particular, public investment in health systems and the willingness of governments to invest in health become key parameters of whether institutions are available to respond to pandemics. The classed nature of health systems means that there are marked differences between survival for different groups of individuals even when other individual differences are accounted for. In addition, the 'inverse care law' means that more vocal, middle-class, sectors of a population are more likely to benefit from health care. Similarly, *preparedness advice* is often written from a perspective that does not take into account material inequalities in society and individuates responsibility for suffering. In examining these processes (Preston 2012, 2019a) concepts of *tacit intentionality* and *path dependency* have been used to explain

© The Author(s) 2020
J. Preston, R. Firth, *Coronavirus, Class and Mutual Aid in the United Kingdom*,
https://doi.org/10.1007/978-3-030-57714-8_3

how inequalities of class, race, gender and other social characteristics have been encoded in preparedness documents and policies. The creation of preparedness policies, many of which are informed by seemingly neutral scientific evidence, occurs in a UK policy environment where most of the politicians and civil servants involved are from a middle-class, often privately educated, background. Sometimes there is a real attempt to engage with issues of social inequality by these groups but the tendency is for issues of class to be neglected in creating 'normative advice' (Preston 2012). Issues of class are referred to as 'indicators or deprivation' or 'socio-economic status' and are considered as 'behavioural characteristics' rather than constructed through structural inequalities. Additionally, there is significant path dependency in preparedness advice as institutions become locked into patterns of behaviour that reproduce similar advice and guidance over time (Preston et al. 2014). For example, in Japan preparedness advice has historically been led by the government with an emphasis on lifelong learning whereas in New Zealand advice is grounded in grassroots communities and local authorities. In the UK, increased centralisation by the Civil Service and the professionalisation of emergency management tend to produce preparedness advice and guidance that is produced under conditions of state centralisation and secrecy. Advice is gradually revealed to the population in what has been referred to as 'surge pedagogy' (Preston 2012). The government issues advice in 'surges' of information rather than as a fully explained narrative arc.

One of these pedagogical surges occurred on 10th March 2020 where the main advice issued to the population in the UK was guidance on handwashing in a series of short, silent, low-budget films which were infrequently broadcast on television and disseminated in social media. This was expanded throughout March and April into a series of public information films and then to the 'stay home', lockdown advice, which in May became 'stay alert'. These were primarily low-key interventions. Preparedness in the UK is not a societal spectacle, as in the United States, but rather a matter of expertly constructed secretive decisions by those who know the 'science' best in terms of the 'models'. Tacit intentionality and path dependence operate together to produce a 'locked in' form of preparedness advice where it is extremely difficult to move preparedness towards a form which takes into account material inequalities and concerns of social and economic justice (Preston 2012, 2019a). Preparedness acts as a form of state survival primarily for the state and capital as abstract entities and the ruling class as their human entities (Preston 2019a).

When preparedness advice moves in the direction of more socially just forms or away from centralising trends (where that is the institutional norm) vested interests and locked in institutional structures tend to pull this back to what were standard practices and there is a low level of innovation in this field. Leaflets and messaging tend to be similar across different crises and standardised messages perpetually repeated in emergencies over time. In the case of COVID-19, for example, the UK's advice is similar to previous campaigns in pandemics, particularly influenza, in terms of hand washing and social distancing which are disseminated through leaflets and public information campaigns. Even the ways in which information is portrayed is similar to previous public information campaigns from the last half century (Preston 2012). In public information films airing on UK television from 18th March 2020, for example, the advice to 'Protect yourself, others and the NHS' was contained in a square similar to that used to signal atomistic (familial) preparedness for previous extreme threats such as the circle containing the 'nuclear family' in the 'Protect and Survive' public information films (Preston 2012). The advice was given by an 'official' in a suit and tie (in this case the Chief Medical Officer) echoing decades of UK public information. Advice and information are given late in the cycle of escalation in 'surge pedagogy' as last minute education close to the peak of the crisis. This lack of consistent and timely information led to widespread confusion over practices such as mask wearing, social distancing and returning to work when the 'stay alert' policy was suddenly revealed in May without a corresponding public information campaign. Alternatives to this established mode of public information, such as memetic forms of advertising and more technological solutions to preparedness information (such as the use of mobile or GPS technologies which are utilised in South Korea), were not being deployed in the UK in the early stages of the pandemic. COVID-19 preparedness operated in the UK, and continues to operate, like a game between the state which holds a hidden 'model' of what might happen next and the public who were drip fed information and advice at times and at a pace that is set by the government. Sometimes the UK population was ahead of the state in terms of 'staying in place' and in a free-market, neo-liberal economy the population will sometimes take actions counter to the government's planning. For example, advice to the population to avoid panic buying may produce the opposite impact as the population may (rightly) perceive this to be a signal that supplies are running short.

In order to consider the neo-liberal approach of the UK government we will first discuss the behavioural science advice before turning to specific elements of this such as quarantine and how these assume a particular approach to class and class strategies privileging middle-class modes of self-making and working. It must be noted that although the UK is formed of separate nations (England, Scotland, Wales and Northern Ireland) in this analysis we will be primarily concerned with the scientific/behavioural advice which is created centrally as part of SAGE (Scientific Advisory Group for Emergencies) and although there may be nuanced differences between the devolved administration there is little substantive difference (as yet) in terms of broad adherence to the central advice. As the pandemic progresses, we might start to see increased divergence. For example, on 10th May there was a clear difference between nations with England changing advice to 'Stay Alert' and other nations (particularly Scotland) sticking to the 'Stay Home' advice.

Nudging the Pandemic: The Neo-Liberal Assumptions of Behavioural Science for Disasters

On 3rd February 2020 the prime minister flanked by his Chief Scientific Officer, Sir Patrick Vallance and his Chief Medical Officer Sir Chris Whitty, gave an account of the COVID-19 action plan. This was one of the first public statements of our pandemic policy. During this press conference we heard that the NHS may have to cancel non-essential operations and that the police may only be able to deal with serious crimes as they would need to concentrate on maintaining social order. The prime minister, Boris Johnson, was, at that point, still openly shaking hands with people on coronavirus wards and boasting about it in public speeches. Perhaps the arrogance of the ruling class is that they feel that germs don't actually impact them although the prime minster was to eventually catch the virus. Aside from that there were no real surprises in terms of the advice possibly because we were at what was called the 'contain' stage of the outbreak. On 12th March 2020 the prime minister gave another press conference starting with an extraordinary but prescient statement that 'It is going to spread further and I must level with you, I must level with the British public: many more families are going to lose loved ones before their time'. The press conference did not announce changes to policy and unlike most other developed countries that had been impacted by the virus there were no announcements of school closures or social distancing measures at that point. Rather, the advice was that people should 'self-isolate' if they have symptoms of the virus (a fever and/or new persistent cough symptoms). This approach was (initially) laissez-faire compared to that of other countries in East Asia (particularly China, Hong Kong and Singapore) and Europe (Italy, Germany and France) and even when compared to some cities in the United States which adopted more extreme social distancing and closure measures. Expectations were that the UK government had a strategy of allowing the pandemic to run through the population to build up what is called 'herd immunity' to the virus. Boris Johnson stated that one theory was in fact for us to 'take it on the chin' in terms of letting the virus attack the population (Hunter 2020). There are eugenic undertones in this idea that the UK population as a whole should act as a buffer to acquire 'herd immunity' and there was a highly negative reaction to this policy. A commentary reported by the *Sunday Times* on the 23rd of March summarised that the views of the prime minister's chief advisor, Dominic Cummings, was along the lines that the policy should be 'herd immunity, protect the economy, and if that means some pensioners die, too bad' (Cummings and Downing Street have since strongly denied that this took place). Other than scientific reasons why herd immunity might not work (that there is no existing immunity to the virus the progression of which is largely unknown and which might dangerously evolve) in getting to herd immunity, without social distancing measures, there would be a large number of unmitigated deaths and serious illnesses. This was such an extraordinary sacrifice that Hunter (2020) reported that some epidemiologists considered that the UK strategy was not serious and some thought that it might be an example of British 'satire'. 'Herd immunity' involves the targeting and dehumanising of whole populations to become a 'herd' (Pilgrim 2008) for the protection of the greater good (in eugenic terms the 'prime' genetic stock) with some very vulnerable people being 'cocooned' or 'shielded' inside their homes. In the context of COVID-19 the population 'herd' of this year's pandemic were implicitly asked to take part in sacrificial action so that future economic and social prosperity could be secured. In any case, the UK's approach to lockdown was to enforce this much later and less strictly than in most other countries. This advice was very different from the advice of other national governments and it is worthwhile to contextualise why the UK government was, overtly or tacitly, adopting this approach in terms of the ways in which 'states of exception' have been used experimentally in this country.

It is not alarmist to state that the UK government has always prepared to take risks with working-class lives experimentally in 'states of emergency' (Preston 2009). Agamben's (2005) 'State of Exception' is frequently seen to be a governmental paradox whereby the state suspends its own laws by legal means in order to create a suspension of democracy and liberty in favour of state sovereignty. One understated feature of the exception is that it also allows for experiments with new forms of governance and rule. The experimental nature of the 'state of exception' is evidenced in plans for 'continuity of government' particularly in the Cold War. In the UK, for example, Cold War plans for national continuity involved experimenting with regional government in a series of 'small states' and fundamental changes to the judicial system involving the suspension of the ordinary legal process as a 'collapsible state' (Preston 2009). It is easy to underestimate the extent to which the UK government is prepared to go to exercise sovereignty in extraordinary situations and the enthusiasm of the state for the suspension of democratic processes in a crisis (Preston 2019b). The novel coronavirus is one such instance where extraordinary state powers and experimental conditions are being used.

These powers are often supported by reference to scientific expertise. In the 'coronavirus crisis' there is a consistent reference to 'the science' by government, particularly regarding behavioural science advice. The prime minister is nearly always joined by the Chief Scientific Officer and the Chief Medical Officer in press conferences and they frequently refer to 'behavioural science' in their statements. Although the government is quite happy to talk about 'science' and 'the science' as if it were unambiguous the behavioural science chosen is selective. This is partly pragmatic as there is no way that all the behavioural science relevant to the topics of pandemic, quarantine and social distancing can be included. If you can change the experts then you can change the advice. The UK government filters its access to behavioural science advice through experts who are selected to be part of SAGE (Scientific Advisory Group for Emergencies). The nature of these meetings is largely conducted in conditions of secrecy and advice is frequently redacted. No such advice can be neutral and free of certain biases, as the members of SAGE would probably accept, but the government selects advice in ways that are both ideological and experimental. For UK academics, there is an implicit tendency to influence government to produce funded 'impact' so there is an incentive to select their own studies and work in doing so. Additionally, there is a constant demand to be experimental and innovative in thinking. This 'thinking differently' about population behaviour is a legacy of the way in which organisations such as the RAND corporation encouraged thinking about disasters but has been advocated by the prime minister's special advisor, Dominic Cummings. The ways in which the UK government traditionally encourages thinking about 'behavioural science' are prone to bias as civil servants inevitably select experts who are 'like them' or part of their social capital network but are also subject to the cult of 'cleverness' in terms of the 'maverick genius', often political advisers, who support the counter-intuitive. In the case of the behavioural science adopted by the UK in the current pandemic this is sometimes influenced by nudge theory, the idea of changing incentives incrementally as the population might become 'tired' of protective measures which can then be put in practice when the crisis peaks. There is also a fear of social disorder which is akin to 'elite panic' in which elites perceive the population as a whole as potentially chaotic and violent in the absence of strong control or incentives (Clarke and Chess 2008). The influence of what has been called the 'Nudge Unit' in influencing the Cabinet Office and the role of selectively chosen behavioural science more generally is implicated in these policies. Alongside the need for 'innovation' and 'new thinking' this has significantly promoted the role of behavioural science to an important part of the process of pandemic management.

The language used to describe the population in some of the more brutal discourses of behavioural science acts to deprive them of agency and humanity. As a 'herd' (in terms of 'herd immunity' or in terms of 'mass population response') the population uses their humanity as a buffer and becomes equivalent to a vector through which the virus passes or a behavioural object to be prodded. The eugenic connotations of this have already been remarked upon but this discourse also massifies the population into a lump of resource that is able to prevent the illness of others. The absence in this portrayal is the 'non-herd' or the 'owners' or 'non-cattle' meaning presumably the ruling class or elites. Erica Lagalisse (2019) in a wide-ranging work on conspiracy theories argues that 'fans' of conspiracies are affectively/emotionally invested in understanding the structures that oppress them, even though their intellectual investment does not identify the same structures of oppression as the intellectual Left. It is not a large leap of political imagination to compare the 'herd' depiction of the UK government with the paranoid and survivalist eagerness with which some conspiracists seek to distinguish themselves from the state's understanding and treatment of individuals as 'sheeple' (a word combining both sheep and people). Relatedly, the idea that the population would become tired of protective measures and the portrayal of them as being influenced by nudges and incentives does not afford them a sense of agency. Rather the 'herd' (even if herd immunity is not used in its biological sense) appears to be an unthinking mass who can be 'stimulated' by incentives from the state. The role of reflexivity, or inter-play, between the state and the population is absent from this discourse. The idea of the herd is in a dynamic with other forms of classed portrayal. Whether 'herd immunity' is explicitly mentioned by government or not, the discourse of government 'science' is to present the working class, particularly, as a non-agentic 'lump' who can be exposed to the virus at work or in their 'dangerous' consumption practices. Against the idea of a 'herd', which is a classed way of considering the way in which the population is comprised, is the conception of a middle-class subject of preparedness who is involved in the making of the self 'above the herd'. Middle-class reflexivity and economic resources, the ability to work from home consistently, to make judgements of those who have to use public transport for work in a pandemic and to obtain consistent home deliveries become a privileged viewpoint in the pandemic. These forms of middle-class subjectivity are implicit in forms of behavioural science research as will be discussed below.

Behavioural Science and Class in the Pandemic

Behavioural science for disasters is a multi-disciplinary field which has been drawn together from primarily disciplinary fields of psychology and sociology that have become fused together in more recent years (Preston 2019a). The naming of this area as 'scientific' is problematic in terms of predicting large-scale societal behaviour in a pandemic as opposed to individual and community behaviour. The focus on 'behaviour' privileges an approach that focuses on the observable rather than on mental, psychoanalytic, psychosocial constructs or on societal concepts. The emphasis is therefore descriptively positivist rather than realist or phenomenological but although the term 'science' implies a positivist approach in reality the body of research in behavioural science is an aggregated body of (often small-scale) studies that are used selectively in terms of what the authorities consider to be of most utility at that time. From a sociological perspective, the ways in which knowledge is used are an important aspect of considering what 'behavioural science' is and how it is employed in a pandemic situation.

The current behavioural science models currently employed to tackle COVID-19 by the UK government do not explicitly refer to social, and certainly not societal, characteristics preferring the term 'heterogeneous populations' (Michie 2020). They also use an individualised model of behaviour which does not take into account material constraints. In terms of hand-washing and other preventative behaviours, for example, the 'COM-B' model is used which refers to Capability, Opportunity and Motivation being combined to produce the required behaviour (Michie 2020). The COM-B model makes assumptions about material resources and social contexts which people require to deal successfully with COVID-19. It also makes broader assumptions concerning the ability of people to navigate and self-manage the epidemic which are heavily classed. In terms of material resources, for example, it requires that individuals 'Ensure ready access to soap and water or alcohol-based (60%+) sanitiser at all times, carry moisturiser if you are concerned about dry hands, make sure you have clean tissues readily available and use household disinfectant to wipe at-risk surfaces' (Michie 2020). The pandemic requires resourced self-management. The use of tissues, and the ways in which they are a middle-class affectation, has been remarked on by Bourdieu as a mode of class distinction. For the middle classes the containment of bodily functions, such as sneezing or laughter, in an unobtrusive way, is key to the making of distinctions:

> It would be easy to show, for example, that Kleenex tissues, which have to be used delicately, with a little sniff from the tip of the nose, are to the big cotton handkerchief, which is blown into sharply and loudly, with the eyes closed and the nose held tightly, as repressed laughter is to a belly laugh, with wrinkled nose, wide-open mouth and deep breathing ('doubled up with laughter'), as if to amplify to the utmost an experience which will not suffer containment, not least because it has to be shared, and therefore clearly manifested for the benefit of others. (Bourdieu 2010, 190)

COM-B also makes middle-class assumptions concerning self-management and reflexivity that assume a middle-class form of cultural capital. When navigating social situations it advises us 'When acceptable ask for and give feedback when you and others are touching mouth / nose / eyes' (Michie 2020). This assumes that personal conduct is a matter of individual policing and social closure and that it is acceptable to comment on the (apparently vulgar and dangerous) behaviour of others whilst learning to correct one's own behaviour. Similarly, the (good) advice not to shake hands is followed by 'explain why you are not engaging in close contact greeting to make it normal and acceptable' (Michie 2020). There are also references to planning that assumes that people have a degree of agency and control in managing their work and informal contacts. People are advised to 'Plan work, travel or recreational activities that do not involve physical social gatherings…Develop explanations for people as to why you are avoiding social gatherings…Plan for practicalities of managing everyday life (e.g. medicines, food, communications)…Plan for financial and social support during isolation' (Michie 2020). If the behavioural science is really for a 'heterogeneous population' it is a 'heterogeneously middle class' population with the ability to plan everyday existence and work so that working from home and avoiding the social world are matters of personal navigation rather than structurally necessary activity. It assumes a middle-class self (Skeggs 2013) that can be bounded and can isolate itself from society whilst policing the boundaries of others through verbal advice to refrain from vulgar activities of self-touching. This is far from the reality of those who care for others (particularly children and older people) as part of the formal and informal economy where boundaries of self/other cannot be planned or predicted. Those working in sectors such as catering/bar work, health services, construction, assembly work and packing/logistics/delivery would find it impossible to 'plan' their own work around lack of contact or to work from home. The self that is assumed here is a reflexive self that can take itself out of society and relations with others. It is:

> …a self that reflects upon itself, simultaneously *externalising itself from social relations* so that the former can reflect and plan its future actions and then reinsert itself back into society through internalization: it is a self that therefore knows itself. (Skeggs 2013, 53, *my italics*)

In the case of the COVID-19 pandemic, a middle-class self is assumed that can literally remove itself from society, carrying a consistently restocked supply of tissues and cleansers, avoiding work (at least work that involves going outside or working with others), touch and sociality and issuing a commentary on the behaviour of others whilst policing the boundaries of the self. The 'working class self' who does not have a personal supply of sanitiser, does not ask for or give comment on other's behaviour, uses public transport and works in occupations that involve no social distancing is depicted as 'excess, waste, disgust' (Skeggs 2013, 99). The supposedly neutral 'science' works as a class strategy of working-class elimination. On the level of individualised social and behavioural science this advice appears to be optimised and correct but it does not consider the material and cultural nature of the majority of people's lives and makes classed assumptions concerning the nature of working lives, self-management, presentation of self and policing the lives of others. In contrast to the behaviour of the (whether explicitly mentioned or not) 'herd' who are considered to be non-agentic and biological 'fodder' that are used to develop 'immunity' in the wider population (particularly in terms of distinguishing between those who need to return to work against those who can work from home) the behavioural science advice privileges the making of a middle-class self who is resource rich and who is in the process of self-making. Therefore, we can see differences in the models that are assumed for middle-class individuals compared to the 'masses'. On the one hand, the COM-B model is a reasonably sophisticated and variegated model of behaviour that has a range of possible outcomes and behaviours that an individual can master (and the emphasis is on the basis of individualised behaviour rather than community actions). On the other hand, the conception of those who do not fall into that category become the subjects of a 'non-model' in terms of behavioural science which does not imply any particular aspect of behaviour. Rather through social 'milling' immunity, or simply increased disease, is experienced by the working-class herd with the cost to the herd being those who are lost. The two models have different necropolitical implications. The survivor is interpellated as agentic, involved in telling of the self and telling others, whereas the victim is described as dangerous to others (through perhaps the necessity of work in contact with others) and as a social 'mass'. With these principles in mind, we will now examine three parts of collective behaviour that have been emphasised in the UK government's behavioural science advice and general guidance: the rationality of 'panic buying', the natural outbreak of 'altruism' and the necessity of social distancing or 'quarantine'.

Panic Buying and the Market

In late March 2020 behaviour inspired by the virus led to shortages in UK supermarkets and other shopping outlets. Images of supermarket shelves that were cleared of stock proliferated on social media. Stocks of toilet paper and hand sanitiser were being rapidly depleted on a daily basis and this seemed to be the initial focus of the panic buying. There were reports on social media that the crisis had resulted in sellers, both online and in shops, selling products at hugely inflated prices, such as £10 for four toilet rolls and £20 for a bottle of hand sanitiser. Other products were also impacted and there were shortages of certain goods including tinned goods, pasta and rice and bottled water which quickly developed into the widespread purchasing of nearly all fresh foodstuffs in supermarkets including fresh meat, milk and fruit and vegetables. This rapid purchasing put pressure on UK supply chains, including warehouses, and meant that workers in the NHS and older, vulnerable adults found that when they could get to supermarkets the shelves were empty of a number of products. This led to a later policy of food parcels being delivered to vulnerable groups by the army and volunteers.

There are two sides to the government advice and use of behavioural science on purchasing. In the press conferences held by Boris Johnson and the Chief Scientific Adviser and Chief Medical Officer panic buying was frequently referred to explicitly in that people should not panic buy but that what appears to be panic buying is a *rational response*. It is those elements of panic and rationality that are classed.

In market logics, the way in which consumers are behaving in 'panic buying' is clearly rational. Unlike the ruling class the purchasing power of those who work and who do not have high levels of savings is regulated in weekly or monthly payments. In practice, this means that shopping is an activity that is scheduled by the arrival of the paycheque or pay in their account. The initial guidance for self-isolation (in terms of those in a household where one member of the household shows symptoms) was extended to *twelve weeks* for those who are over the age of 70 or who have underlying health conditions and by March the whole population was in 'lockdown'. Under these circumstances people will rationally decide to purchase not only to stockpile food and sanitary products for times of isolation but also to avoid future shortages and price rises. It is rational to buy now, and more than you would normally, if it will simply not be available in the future.

Stockpiling, what is called panic buying, even grabbing toilet rolls from the shelves, therefore makes sense in behavioural science if we accept the neo-liberal nature of the ways in which markets operate with atomistic consumers acting in their own self interests. In its own terms, as a capitalist logic, this makes sense but neglects the social and classed nature of markets, particularly in terms of inequality. As we considered earlier, commodity production is classed and that for the ruling class their markets are perceptually absent from the rest of society. The ruling class have an expectation that their food will arrive at the table and that their fridges will be fully stocked as they employ a retinue of chefs, servants and sommeliers who source their meals for them. The ruling class exist in a strange form of utopian socialism, being free from want or necessity. In an example of this, the Queen of England went into social isolation in the week of the 16th March as an 'example' to the nation. The 'example' is only possible given the extraordinary wealth of the Queen whereas those who have to hunt for reasonably priced toilet roll cannot set an 'example' and are positioned as vulgar consumers.

Aside from the ruling class where markets are invisible to the majority, the market as played out on supermarket shelves *appears* to be fair (in that every consumer is treated equally when it comes to price) but masks obvious inequalities. Firstly, markets are exclusionary in terms of entry costs. For example, Ocado (a delivery firm that markets itself primarily to middle-class consumers) which was reporting high demand for their home delivery service in the pandemic has a minimum shop of £40 and in late March 2020 closed the availability of delivery slots to new consumers. Secondly, one of the basic principles of economics is that demand is only actualised if it is *effective demand*. If people don't have the income then they cannot participate in purchasing. As has been previously explained, most 'big shops' for households peak around pay days. Thirdly, panic buying spikes demand and prices rise particularly for people who have to wait to purchase or who cannot gain access to a wide variety of suppliers. So 'panic-buying' is depicted is a *classed activity* that might be avoided if a household has the spare income, travel or access to home delivery. Market rationality excuses inequality in ability to respond to a pandemic. Using purchasing power and mobility to elbow out the working classes from the toilet roll aisles through home deliveries in an exclusive consumer club is only rational in an irrational economic system. For those who can get to the supermarkets on low incomes it does make sense to buy now as they can not necessarily rely on the state to support them.

The ways in which this sort of purchasing has been portrayed in the media have also been classed. It is those working-class consumers who have to raid the shelves for the last supplies of hand sanitiser who are portrayed as excessive and vulgar rather than the middle-class Waitrose 'prepper' who can fill their car with shopping. Bourdieu (2010, 71) refers to the importance of the 'mode of acquisition' as a feature of class distinction. Although the working and middle class have identical bodily functions and often consume the same products consumption is seen to be 'vulgar' if it is excessive and visible. Hence some elements of the bourgeois middle classes during the crisis could gain cultural capital by making their consumption worthy and unnoticeable through buying upcycled materials and raw foodstuffs. In a pandemic, cultural capital may be gained through disassociation from 'vulgar' panic buying which is seen as a socially denigrated 'mode of acquisition'. Similarly, construction workers were, at the end of March, being judged as not following rules for social distancing on construction sites rather than questions being raised about the necessity of building luxury flats and apartments in a pandemic. By the end of April, construction workers had the second highest death rate amongst men from coronavirus throughout England and Wales (ONS 2020), the first being security guards who also work in construction as well as hospitals. As considered in the first chapter, members of the ruling class seem to be entirely absent from perceptual realms of consumption and production, accessing private islands and mainland, guarded, retreats. As such the judgement of taste falls on those whose consumption or production is most visible.

Altruism and Pro-Social Behaviour

In the 3rd February prime ministerial press conference it was stated that behavioural science research showed that COVID-19 will bring about an 'outbreak' of altruism. There are many opportunities for mutual aid, even in a pandemic, but to use altruism as a stop gap for a state that will withdraw health and public protection (already under pressure and unequally distributed) is a way of managing disaster capitalism. Again, what many behavioural science models of altruism in disasters neglect is the economic and political contexts of disasters. In previous work (Preston et al. 2014) we looked at these contexts for community mutual aid in what was called an 'ecological' (in terms of social, not natural ecologies) model of disaster response. Across five countries (UK, United States, Japan, New Zealand and Germany) it was found that all disasters involve mutual aid and altruism but where there is extreme inequality in response the disaster is reframed and mutual aid is politicised. New Zealand farmers have been known to steal generators to benefit their rural communities, unemployed Japanese young people set up their own online disaster advice from their bedrooms and British villages organise their own flood defences and express anger at politicians who visit following flood events. In the United States, in Hurricane Sandy, mutual aid became a concern for the Occupy movement (which renamed itself 'Occupy Sandy') and communities, that were incensed at how the geographies of disaster relief meant that the state prioritised middle-class communities for recovery. In considering altruism in its economic and political contexts it is important to consider how these actions can be appropriated by the state. For example, an emphasis on developing a test for those who have developed antibodies to COVID-19 rather than for those who are currently sick due to the illness is so that the government can 'mobilise' both volunteers and workers to facilitate rapid economic regeneration. The state attempts to depoliticise mutual aid by ignoring these activist aspects in its interpretations of behavioural science. These arguments, concerning the state appropriation of mutual aid, are explored in the next chapter.

Self-Isolation and Quarantine

In the UK at the start of the pandemic there was guidance on how people should 'self-isolate' if they, or any member of their family, have symptoms of the virus. This eventually became displaced by the advice to 'stay at home' for all households. At the outset, it should be said that the original guidance for self-quarantine in terms of COVID-19 was, from an epidemiological perspective, good advice as this can prevent the spread of the pandemic and 'flatten the curve' in terms of decreasing the burden on the NHS. However, in the UK the advice on how to self-isolate following exposure to COVID-19 made extraordinary assumptions about how most people actually live and exposed how the state tends to think about working-class people more generally.

The original guidance on quarantine in the UK for COVID-19 was the Public Health England factsheet 'Advice Sheet—Home Isolation' (Gov.UK 2020) which was the active advice before 12th March 2020. Subsequent to this there was a slight 'recalibration' of the advice but this was mainly in terms of accepting that some people would not be able to follow this advice, and suggesting mitigations that they could take, rather than aiming at addressing some of the material disadvantages. On 23rd March the UK was placed in full 'lockdown' under the 'stay at home' guidance, supported by legislation. Despite the changes, considering the original advice is instructive as it provides an insight into the ways in which the UK government initially considered self-isolation prior to criticisms by other political parties and the press.

The advice in the online resource in early March was called 'Stay At Home' which is a familiar phrase from UK public information going back at least to the 1970s. For example, in the 'Protect and Survive' public information films from the 1970s which were designed to mitigate against the impact of thermonuclear war 'stay at home' was also the message, prioritising the safety and security of individuals as part of a nuclear family. In this case, isolation seems to be good advice in terms of mitigating against the spread of a virus (and ostensibly protecting individuals and families) but this depends on their access to home delivery and safety at home. However, this advice not only has unfortunate echoes of previous public information films and booklets but also of recent contexts where 'stay put' had horrific consequences. Namely, in the Grenfell Tower fire in June 2017 in which seventy-two people were killed, and many more seriously injured, in a tower block fire the policy 'stay put' was in place. The 'stay put' policy, alongside what were well noted (by the residents) alleged failures in the building construction and safety measures, was thought to be responsible for the disaster (Preston 2019a). In these circumstances 'Rather than seeing "stay put" as objective and technical advice it is best seen as a social technology. "Stay put" has historically been used for social reasons in terms of the State meeting its strategic objectives whilst keeping populations inert' (Preston 2019a, 48). The indeterminacy of the 'stay put' advice (in Grenfell it was qualified with various statements around how to observe this policy) meant that the responsibility for survival is passed on to the subjects of the advice rather than the state. This leads to questioning whether this advice should be followed or not which was even expressed by politicians. For example, the British MP Jacob Rees-Mogg, Leader of the House of Commons, expressed his disbelief that anyone would follow official advice in these circumstances and stated that people who do so were lacking 'common sense'. The experience of Grenfell, and these comments, suggests that following official advice to remain in place is not necessarily the correct thing to do, particularly for working-class residents. Therefore, the advice to 'stay put' or 'stay home' in the UK in 2020 takes place within a particular social and cultural context where trust in official advice of this type may be questioned by working-class people. Grenfell Tower provides a hugely symbolic recent reminder on the way that official advice to stay where you are can act as eliminationism.

In this context where 'stay put' has a social history, the willingness of the population to follow guidance might be questioned given that official advice has not always been the best advice. This was certainly the case on the weekend of 21st and 22nd March where a number of members of the public attended parks, markets and seaside towns which led to a 'lockdown' of the majority of the UK population on 23rd March with draconian restrictions on public behaviour (allowing exercise only once a day and enforcing that people should only leave their homes for essential work or medical/food visits).

Turning to the initial advice for COVID-19 quarantine, like all UK government public information, the factsheet starts with some knowing advice from the state in terms of what might have been previously described as 'advice for the householder' in the Cold War:

> Your local health protection team and your doctor have agreed that you may stay at home while you wait for the results of tests for COVID-19 (SARS-CoV-2) infection. This is because you do not need to be admitted to hospital and because you have agreed to follow the important instructions described below. (GOV.UK 2020)

This is an important statement as it makes a covert reference to the power of the state to impose quarantine. You are staying at home because you have agreed to follow the (pro-active health) advice otherwise the state can use its powers to impose quarantine on you. This raises interesting questions about whether the guidance, or support available, actually enables people to abide by this guidance and how powers might be used to enforce this. At the end of March 2020 there was an indication that the police (or other agents of the state) might be allowed to use powers of detention and arrest for those who did not maintain quarantine and in April there were arrests and fines for those not following the subsequent 'lockdown' advice. Therefore, although the advice is badged as guidance, the guidance is backed by the power of the state to enforce, through the removal of other rights, what is advised.

The guidance then discusses how quarantine might be practised:

> You should stay in a well-ventilated room with a window to outside that can be opened, separate from other people in your home. Keep the door closed. Use a separate bathroom from the rest of the household, if available. If you have to share these facilities, regular cleaning will be required. (GOV.UK 2020)

There are assumptions about where people live and what they are able to do in this statement. Having a well-ventilated room, with a window and a separate bathroom seems to imply that a person will be living in private accommodation with a window and an *en suite* bathroom or perhaps two bathrooms. The assumption that the accommodation has these facilities, and is not over-occupied, makes classed judgements about how quarantine is conducted as a social practice. There are obviously material differences implied in the quarantine advice but this also extends to practices and time regimes. As the guidance continues, if separate bathroom facilities are not available then there is advice about regular cleaning, bathroom rotas and separate towels. This emphasis on rotas and regular cleaning implies that there is an optimised model of care and cleaning that it is possible to impose on a household. This infers that there are 'ways' of cleaning as there are 'ways of cooking' (Bourdieu 2010, 18) that represents the proper way that household management should be practiced. This makes bourgeois assumptions concerting organisation and communal living which requires space and resources. In terms of childcare or looking after an elderly relative or extended family member it assumes that the household is able to isolate and routinise care. This privileges ideas of 'separateness' and 'self-making' in middle-class households and is hostile to ideas of care and touch. As Skeggs (1997) states:

> The working class are never free from the judgements of imaginary and real others that position them, not just as different, but as inferior, as inadequate. Homes and bodies are where respectability is displayed but where class is lived out as the most omnipresent form, engendering surveillance and constant assessment of themselves. these areas where taste operates to commit symbolic violence. (Skeggs 1997, 90)

In this case, the 'imaginary other' of the official advice means that working-class selves are judged as inferior for following 'dangerous practices' of care. Hence processes of care, touch and sharing are denaturalised as harmful and contaminating of others. As Skeggs states, following Bourdieu, this is not just a form of labelling but symbolic violence, a denigration of working-class resources. This enables the working class to be labelled as a 'threat' to society for not following the guidelines. However, the idea that children, or other members of the family, might be isolated if they had symptoms of COVID-19 is simply not tenable for many households. Similarly, despite the (seemingly good) advice not to invite people into one's home this contradicts the earlier advice concerning mutual aid. It is not clear how working-class single parent households would be able to cope with a COVID-19 infection if they and their child are both suffering otherwise:

> Only those who live in your home should be allowed to stay. Do not invite or allow visitors to enter. If you think there is an essential need for someone to visit, then discuss it with your designated medical contact first. If it is urgent to speak to someone who is not a member of your household, do this over the phone. (GOV.UK 2020)

There is also an expectation that food will be available for the period of quarantine. Originally the suggestion was that quarantine was followed for 14 days for families, or individuals living together, that needed to self-isolate, which would extend for a further 7 days if there was an individual that had symptoms since then. As of Monday 23rd March the whole population of the UK was asked to self-isolate only leaving the house for exercise (once a day), for medical or food supplies or for work where it was not possible to work from home and not to invite visitors into the home (which restricts the scope of mutual aid). Moreover, those who had underlying health conditions were asked to isolate for twelve weeks. For those with underlying health conditions, provision of food supplies was accounted for (with army and volunteer logistics potentially delivering food). There is a huge disconnect between this advice and the levels of food poverty and food insecurity in the UK. As the advice states:

> You will need to ask for help if you require groceries, other shopping or medications. Alternatively, you can order by phone or online. The delivery instruction needs to state that the items are to be left outside, or in the porch, or as appropriate for your home. (GOV.UK 2020)

In China and Hong Kong the use of delivery services of the Deliveroo and Uber Eats variety became increasingly popular due to quarantine. Similarly, the UK government was allowing the *market* to respond to fulfil the demand for online shopping by considering whether supermarkets should be freed from restrictions under competition policy and allowing them to make deliveries twenty-four hours a day. The pandemic therefore leads to a relaxation of the rules of how some capitals (businesses) operate and compete whilst closing some companies (such as pubs, restaurants and cafes). However, references to home delivery and the need to purchase face-masks and cleaning substances make it clear that this is a period of isolation that requires economic resources and stockpiling.

It should be noted that the advice was slightly updated on 12th March 2020 as the UK government advice changed so that those who thought they were displaying symptoms should self-isolate for seven days. The amendments to the guidance did begin to take into account some of the socially unjust features of the above advice. Eventually the UK government made the whole household the 'unit' of protection with the 'Stay Home' advice although 'households' can differ markedly in terms of structure and number of occupants.

By the time of the UK 'lockdown' the government was starting to show some awareness of the differences in housing tenure by class. However, people were obviously concerned about their elderly relatives who needed care (particularly in care homes where the death rate was particularly high), about the lack of sick pay in their jobs, about living pay cheque to pay cheque and about how to maintain themselves with serious health problems. Of course, this is a class issue and one where the violent and exploitative nature of capitalism is clear. Two million workers who earn less than £118 a week, workers on zero-hours contracts or in the gig economy, those who do not receive sick pay (and there are nearly two million of those) and nearly five million workers who are self-employed including hairdressers and van drivers whose income fluctuates wildly with economic activity were disadvantaged by these policies. Self-isolation and preparing for quarantine are costly activities. The Department of Work and Pensions (DWP) who process benefit payments in the UK did make some ad-hoc provisions for claimants (and the number of claimants is accelerating rapidly as unemployment rises to levels never seen before in the UK) but these still depend on the willingness of 'work coaches' to exercise discretion and it does little to ease the (often substantial) delay between claiming and receiving benefits.

Conclusion

As has been explained in this chapter, behavioural science advice is framed in a neo-liberal context which accepts market logics and privileges middle-class resources and perspectives. In this way the working class are discursively framed as being a 'herd' (even if the term 'herd immunity' is not explicitly used) whose 'othered' positionality and behaviours are facilitating the pandemic. On 22nd March 2020 it was apparent that a large number of people were not following the government advice to socially isolate and avoid social contact as people visited public parks, beaches and shopping centres. In the media reporting of these incidents the working class are portrayed as being a 'threat' to others through their behaviour in the pandemic as caravan holidays, visiting holiday resorts such as Skegness and queueing in supermarkets are classified as threatening and vulgar whereas those who can afford and arrange home deliveries and can take private flights or isolated holidays were not subject to the same classification (although interestingly in a number of regions such as Cornwall and the Highlands the local authorities were critical of those visiting the region who had 'second homes' there and who were seen to be fleeing London).

As McKenzie (2010, 210) states, working-class people are not only demonised but also airbrushed out of UK society by government and media and this also applies to official guidance and how they are portrayed in the pandemic. The working class are being framed in their embodied existence, *as the pandemic itself.* Bizarrely, the living labour that maintains capital is being portrayed as a viral threat to it. This unnatural feature of the pandemic (the destruction of bodies) is actually central to capitalism as it is exclusively interested in the labour power of individuals (an abstract quality in terms of the ability to create value) where concrete labour is almost incidental to the process of value creation. The fact that labour is embodied in a human being with physical and mental capacities is, at some level, repulsive to capital as it has to cajole labour power from a living subject through the payment of a wage in order to create surplus value (Marx 1976). Hence capitalism's relation to the pandemic is both perverse and naturalised as it needs labour power to survive but the bodies that are the carriers of that labour power might contain the virus that might halt production. The emphasis by capitalists on removing people from production throughout its history reaches its apogee in a pandemic where people are removed (sometimes forcibly by the state or through death and incapacity by the virus) but capitalists suddenly realise the importance of workers to their operations (in that not every operation can be mechanised and that the process of mechanisation ultimately leads to falling profits).

The classed (and gendered/raced) aspects and the material nature of people's lives were not part of the behavioural science or government guidance, particularly in the early days of the advice in the UK. These issues are not just considerations of equity but *are* ethical (Butler 2004) and political questions of the deepest kind and also questions in terms of the logic of pandemic preparedness. The state's idea of 'asking for help' is a weak way of phrasing what people in working-class communities do all of the time through mutual aid. We might assume that social forms of 'help' in communities are already being maximised. What it means to be altruistic in a pandemic context needs to be thought through. It would take a particular form of altruism for a working-class community to organise to clean the toilet of an elderly couple where one party suffers from COVID-19, for example as would be implied in the initial guidance. However, forms of mutual aid might arise that do not involve breaking quarantine such as ordering supplies for those who cannot otherwise afford it. Communities might collectively buy, or appropriate in other ways, the resources that they might need and they are already doing this even without COVID-19. As it appears that the economy has come to a 'sudden stop' the state is moving to collectivise the forms of health and care necessary to deal with a pandemic and set up its own form of mutual aid through schemes such as 'NHS volunteers'.

For some, the massive intervention of the UK state in markets, supporting jobs and rent and in logistics, networks and mutual aid suggests some kind of transition to mutualism, or even socialism, in the country. Although there are obvious tendencies towards collectivism, a clearer comprehension of the interconnectedness of society and a moral understanding of the plight of health workers, key workers and the unemployed, the state is not the vehicle to deliver social change. In capitalist societies, the state provides the function of guaranteeing the continuity of capital and has, at its basis, the forms of value generated by workers exploited by capitalism. In previous work the term 'collapsible state' (Preston 2009) has been used to refer to the way in which the state is able to reduce its key functions in a major disaster (such as a pandemic) which can then be re-established after the disaster. Elements of the 'collapsible state' are evident in the current UK strategy for the virus in terms of Continuity of Government (picking a 'designated survivor' in the event that the prime minister is not available and the isolation and protection of the Queen) but to many it would seem as though the state is massively expanding. However, the nature of this expansion is not to socialise the means of production but rather to maintain these means in the hands of capitalists and rentiers whilst providing a 'safety net' to workers to maintain consumption and temporarily pay mortgages and rents. Obviously, there are principles regarding equity within this policy but the criticality of the virus for a capitalist society is the threat that it imposes to the capitalist system rather than the population (Klein 2008). There might be a 'pause' in some elements of capitalist production but this is subsidised by the state as the sovereign consumer. The state is also colonising those elements of mutual aid and social action that existed prior to the pandemic (ironically which previously arose as a result of the absence of the state in public services) which are useful to it in the management of the virus and the continuity of business operations whilst neglecting other functions, such as maintaining food banks. This is the subject of the next chapter which considers the colonisation of mutual aid and the possibility of non-state alternatives to the neo-liberal, classed, management of the pandemic based on anarchist and autonomist principles.

References

Agamben, G. (2005). *State of Exception*. Chicago: University of Chicago Press.
Bourdieu, P. (2010). *Distinction*. London: Routledge.
Butler, J. (2004). *Precarious Life: The Power of Mourning and Violence*. London: Verso.

Clarke, L., & Chess, C. (2008). Elites and Panic: More to Fear than Fear Itself. *Social Forces, 87*(2), 993–1014. https://doi.org/10.1353/sof.0.0155.

GOV.UK. (2020, May 21). *Advice for Home Isolation.* Retrieved from: https://www.gov.uk/government/publications/wuhan-novel-coronavirus-self-isolation-for-patients-undergoing-testing/advice-sheet-home-isolation

Hunter, J. (2020, March). *COVID-19 and the Stiff Upper Lip – The Pandemic Response in the United Kingdom, New England Journal of Medicine.* https://www.nejm.org/doi/full/10.1056/NEJMp2005755?af=R&rss=currentIssue

Klein, N. (2008). *The Shock Doctrine.* London: Penguin.

Lagalisse, E. (2019). *Occult Features of Anarchism: With Attention to the Conspiracy of Kings and the Conspiracy of the Peoples.* London: PM Press.

Marx, K. (1976). *Capital: A Critique of Political Economy, Volume 1.* London: Penguin.

McKenzie, L. (2010). *Getting By: Estates, Class and Culture in Austerity Britain.* Bristol: Policy Press.

Michie, S. (2020, May 21). *Behavioural Science Must Be at the Heart of the Public Health Response to Covid-19.* Retrieved from: https://blogs.bmj.com/bmj/2020/02/28/behavioural-science-must-be-at-the-heart-of-the-public-health-response-to-covid-19/

ONS. (2020). Coronavirus (COVID-19) Related Deaths by Occupation, England and Wales: Deaths Registered Up to and Including 20 April 2020. *Office for National Statistics.* https://www.ons.gov.uk/peoplepopulationandcommunity/healthandsocialcare/causesofdeath/bulletins/coronaviruscovid19relateddeathsbyoccupationenglandandwales/deathsregistereduptoandincluding20april2020. Accessed 11 June 2020.

Pilgrim, D. (2008). The Eugenic Legacy in Psychology and Psychiatry. *International Journal of Social Psychiatry, 54*(3), 272–284. https://doi.org/10.1177/0020764008090282.

Preston, J. (2009). Preparing for Emergencies: Citizenship Education, 'whiteness' and Pedagogies of Security. *Citizenship Studies, 13*(2), 187–200. https://doi.org/10.1080/13621020902731223.

Preston, J. (2012). *Disaster Education: 'Race', Equity and Pedagogy.* Rotterdam: Sense Publishers. 9460918727. 9789460918728.

Preston, J. (2019a). *Grenfell Tower: Preparedness, Race and Disaster Capitalism.* London: Palgrave. 3319968513. 978-3-319-96850-6.

Preston, J. (2019b). Overkill: Why Universities Modelling the Impact of Nuclear War in the 1980s Could Not Change the Views of the Security State. In L. Gearon (Ed.), *The Routledge International Handbook of Universities, Security and Intelligence Studies* (pp. 394–402). London: Routledge.

Preston, J., Chadderton, C., & Kitagawa, K. (2014). The 'State of Exception' and Disaster Education: A Multilevel Conceptual Framework with Implications for Social Justice. *Globalisation, Societies and Education, 12*(4), 437–456. https://doi.org/10.1080/14767724.2014.901906.

Skeggs, B. (1997). *Formations of Class and Gender*. London: Sage.

Skeggs, B. (2013). *Class, Self, Culture*. London: Routledge.

4

Mutual Aid, Anarchist Preparedness and COVID-19

Rhiannon Firth

Introduction

In past decades, we have seen a growing trend for the state to rely on spontaneous community responses to compensate for its growing incapacity and indifference and to manipulate media and social media to relay messages in the interests of repressive social control and behavioural nudging. These dynamics reduce the capacity for social insurrection or revolution and can have a de-radicalising effect on social movements. This chapter considers the perspective of 'disaster anarchism' and the practice of mutual aid disaster relief as an alternative to both market- and state-based preparedness solutions. Mutual aid is a practice of community helping with roots in anarchist though and working-class communities which aims to transgress the hierarchies of established charities and erase distinctions between helpers and helped in order to prefigure a more equal—and stateless—society. However, the practice in its recent incarnation within the COVID-19 crisis appears prone to appropriation by a well-meaning middle class embodying the logic of the state: a depoliticised form of relief and reconstruction that is almost entirely compatible with neoliberal capitalism and its institutions, functioning to restore

J. Preston, R. Firth, *Coronavirus, Class and Mutual Aid in the United Kingdom*,
https://doi.org/10.1007/978-3-030-57714-8_4

'normality' (or an even more terrifying 'new normal') in a context of the withdrawal of state welfare functions. Nevertheless, mutual aid retains an important place within a much broader repertoire of anarchist critique and action. This chapter considers the difference in perspective between the state-centred perspective of mainstream disaster studies, which views human co-operation as an anomaly to be harnessed in the interests of capital, and the anarchist perspective which understands mutual aid as an expression of an authentic 'outside' to relations of hierarchy, competition, control and domination. It is argued that anarchists do not draw distinctions between stages of disasters such as preparedness, relief and recovery; nor do they view disasters as ruptures in the smooth running of things. The essence of the anarchist perspective is an understanding of disasters as constitutive of capitalist inequality and state authoritarianism. This chapter presents an imperative for anarchists to resist the classed colonisation of their movements and the recuperation and co-optation of their radical activities into bureaucratised and regulated forms of 'social capital'. In order to do so, anarchists must maintain radical intentionality at the level of desire, raise consciousness via robust structural critique and create strong links between mutual aid and more confrontational activities that defend communities from dispossession such as strikes and occupations as well as longer-term co-operative infrastructure and permaculture projects.

The Emergence of Disaster Studies: Community Response as 'Post-Disaster Utopia'

The perspective on community response to disasters that dominates disaster studies and mainstream consciousness today dates back to the late 1950s and early 1960s, when North American disaster researchers and media reporters would laud the community action that arose in the immediate aftermath of a 'natural disaster' such as a hurricane, tornado or flood. The term 'post-disaster utopia' was used in early texts to describe a period where feelings of camaraderie and euphoria would lead people to put aside prior differences in order to roll up their sleeves and work together to selflessly help others during the recovery effort (Wolfenstein 1957). One of the first renowned sociologists of disaster, Charles Fritz, argued contrary to others of his era who feared widespread panic and chaos, that large-scale disasters paradoxically appear to produce 'mentally healthy' conditions and that people living in heavily bombed cities in Britain during WWII had 'significantly higher morale' than people living in lighter bombed cities (Fritz 1966: 6). Fritz pre-empts later structuralists by arguing that disasters bring into focus the impact of ongoing systemic crisis on everyday life by erasing the contrast between normal conditions and 'disaster'. In particular, he highlights the failure of modern societies to meet 'human needs for community' (Ibid: 25) and argues that disasters produce a societal shock that helps people to build bonds through shared experiences. Drawing on Fritz, later researchers use the term 'therapeutic community' (Barton 1969). According to these accounts, the 'utopian' period of solidarity, consensus and mutual aid unavoidably recedes after the initial relief efforts as the everyday divisions and differences settle in, at which point it is necessary for a specialised bureaucracy to step in to administer the longer-term tasks of recovery (Erikson 1991). The anthropological/structural approach shows 'disasters do not just happen' (Oliver-Smith and Hoffman 2002) and are compounded by not only human infrastructures but also by political structures and cultural values and norms. However, despite this somewhat relativist stance, these writers view 'post-disaster solidarity' as an almost universal human response, that cannot be explained by rational choice, resource mobilisation or other social movement theories that dichotomise reason and emotion (Oliver-Smith 1999).

These accounts are interesting, because they all link the sociology of disasters to human psychology, pre-empting neoliberal discourses of 'resilience' which mobilise notions of 'emergent togetherness' to place agency and responsibility for recovering from higher-level shocks onto lower-level communities and individuals (Drury et al. 2009). The currently hegemonic public health model is inseparable from disaster management, cybernetic co-ordination and behavioural nudge psychology. This thread was developed by Enrico Quarantelli, a leading name in disaster studies from the late 1970s until the present day. Quarantelli was a student of Fritz, and similarly critiqued the top-down 'command and control' approach to risk management that saw the potential for disaster planning and management to manipulate 'prosocial behaviour' in the interests of restoring 'normalcy' (Quarantelli 1998). Following a cybernetic model which valorises feedback systems he argued that disasters impact differently on different segments of society and communities have their own pre-existing 'patterns of authority' and 'autonomous decision-making' (Ibid: 9) that ought to be left in place. Disaster planning deals with aggregate data and ought to 'focus on general principles and not specific details' (Ibid: 10) and should also 'be vertically and horizontally integrated' (Ibid: 12). This initially gives the appearance of equal treatment and a role for horizontalist organisations such as mutual aid groups. However, the integration of the horizontal with the vertical relies on the planning and management functions of (secretive) state agencies to oversee and co-ordinate their actions in order to differentiate between 'helpful' and injurious emergent actions—and ultimately to use generic structural adjustments, 'education' and 'nudges' to manipulate the beliefs and behaviour of populations in order to encourage those actions that are seen as helpful to the state (see particularly Quarantelli 1998: 12–14). Actions helpful to the state are not judged via democratic means, but rather via the technocratic knowledge of experts (Ibid: 14). While the discourse seems entirely opposed to hierarchical and top-down control, it relies on the same logic of disposability and exclusion of that which is not useful to the state and capitalism. It is problem-solving rather than critical research, and treats humans as outward-directed nodes who can easily change behaviour based on promises of reward or threats of punishment, ignoring complex and often conflicting dynamics of meaning, belief, trust, desire and the unconscious.

Neoliberal State, Capital and Cybernetic Governance

Quarantelli's approach to disaster is located in the context of wider transformation of the relationship between the state and capital that began in the late twentieth century. The early twentieth century saw the rise of

Fordism which is a centralised and organised form of capitalism, based on mass production and consumption, where the state acts as an organiser and stabiliser for capital. In the late twentieth and early twenty-first century, the development of post-Fordist neoliberal capitalism has led the state to significantly relinquish this role, while at the same time, in developed countries, manufacturing has given way to the service economy and more precarious forms of work (Lash and Urry 1987). With the rise of New Public Management from the 1980s onwards, the autonomy of the professional/included stratum in both public and private institutions was largely lost to managerialists, who embodied a state-capitalist logic with decentralised cybernetic components. Rather than acting as rigid Fordist bureaucrats and taking a top-down universalising approach to managing risks, the 'cadres' of 'the new spirit of capitalism' (Boltanski and Chiapello 2005) were trained to build scenario responses to risk in terms of behavioural nudges, proactive measures, quantification and 'flexibility'—which simultaneously fuels uncertainty, insecurity and panic—as well as authoritarianism and top-down control, despite outwardly appearing to resemble decentralised organisation and endowing social actors with a sense of autonomy. There is an issue here, not only that technocratic and managerial authority is undemocratic, but also as revealed by Naomi Klein, the unelected managerial class acts in the interests of capital. Klein coined the term 'disaster capitalism' to refer to the way in which, in all kinds of disasters, powerful people use proxy global recovery agencies at a local level to clear out deprived communities and profitably reconstruct them as neoliberal developments (Klein 2007).

The current public health response to COIVD-19 in the United States and UK might be understood to stem partly from this ethos of population management through micro-political behavioural nudges and incentives, instead of relating to specific individuals with their particular needs (as would be the case in a genuinely decentralised system), or applying general principles (as in a centralised system). In health terms, the shift from Fordist centralised bureaucracy to cybernetic managerialism was reflected in a shift from health as a human right embodied in individuals and enacted (unequally and patchily, but ostensibly universally) through welfare provision to a new discourse of 'public health' focusing on the regulation of aggregates through Foucauldian biopower. This cybernetic view tends to treat the sick as the enemy—or at least as dysfunctional nodes that are disruptive to the functioning of the overall system—to be controlled through authoritarian but decentralised behavioural nudges such as (sometimes vague and confusing) social distancing rules, in which the responsibility for interpreting and successfully following the rules rests with the individual. Take for example the UK government's advice on easing lockdown rules and encouraging a return to work, that individuals ought to 'stay alert' in order to 'control the virus' (Alexander 2020). Health becomes a 'game' which the sick are perceived to have failed—for example the advice to 'wash or sanitise hands frequently' assumes constant access to bathroom facilities, running water and soap which are not always readily available for homeless people for example, and the ability to purchase sanitiser during a panic-buying crisis when prices are exorbitantly inflated. Neoliberal public health emphasises personal responsibility for health outcomes, mimicking a decentralised approach whilst behind the scenes state, military, industrial and pharmaceutical capitalist technocrats are rigging the game to achieve desired (profitable) outcomes.

To complicate matters somewhat, the current conjecture appears to contain social forces towards a gradual discrediting of neoliberal approaches, which is reinforced in the current crisis by the fact that individual health outcomes also affect third parties. This is leading to a resurgence of public health discourses that are basically totalitarian in character; mimicking the increasing securitisation and militarisation of responses to other crises such as the climate-refugee crisis and the increasing bordering of nations. This may be leading to a recomposition of state and capital in new formations that Benjamin Franks calls 'nationalist capitalism' (Franks 2020: 152) and Ian Bruff calls 'authoritarian neoliberalism' (Bruff 2014). There is a new root discourse emerging—away from 'risk management' towards 'new threats' where problems are cast as starting in disorderly zones on the edges of the world system, then filtering inwards, requiring strengthened borders, 'security' and/or neo-colonialism under the guise of 'militant humanitarianism' (Hannigan 2012: 113). Market logic has also devastated the health services in poorer areas of rich countries, so that whereas the margins were once associated with 'tropical' or Third-World areas, one increasingly finds the 'margins' within the core—for example poverty-stricken black communities in post-Katrina New Orleans (Davis 2005). Nevertheless, the new discourse shares the same 'social capital' (Putnam 1993) assumption that the state provides order, cohesion and security to civilised society whilst mobilising its creative energy, and disease and disorder come from a chaotic or barbaric 'outside' or 'elsewhere', in a denial and disavowal of the devastation caused by withdrawing capital, and the knock-on effect for highly interconnected global health outcomes (Davis 2020). This view might be termed 'associationalist' as it assumes that the affairs of society can be managed through voluntary and democratically self-governing associations, and that there is a high degree of complementarity in the association between these groups and the state.

Associationalist views are very prominent in disaster research, the argument usually being that societies with greater social capital are better able to prepare for and mitigate the effects of disasters, and that states can mobilise social capital in their organisation of recovery efforts (e.g. Mathbor 2007; Nakagawa and Shaw 2004; Aldrich 2012). The explicit monetisation of social bonds inherent in the idea of 'social *capital*' coincided with transformations in ideas around the structure and purpose of both left- and right-wing governments in the UK and United States embodied in initiatives like the Obama administration's 'Open Government Initiative' and David Cameron's 'Big Society', both of which encouraged more socially active citizenry and dispersal of information through an ethos of 'transparency' and decentralisation of knowledge, and the 'co-production of government services and democracy' (The Invisible Committee 2014: 103–4). When society and the state are seen as complimentary and mutually supporting, only the sections of 'civil society' that are legible to the state and it can capitalise upon and control are seen as 'social capital'. Other social forces are a threat to be controlled—through recuperation or repression. This links to disaster policy through the idea of 'risk society' (Beck 2002) where the role of the state is to distribute risk in a similar way in which it distributes welfare. This led to a discourse of 'vulnerability' and 'resilience'. These are often seen as conflicting discourses, with 'vulnerability' cast as a social democratic discourse seeking the redistribution of risks and welfare to reduce structural inequalities which unfairly expose poorer, racialised and other marginalised communities to hazard; whereas 'resilience' is associated with smaller government and the privatisation of risk alongside the need for individuals and communities to take responsibility for their own exposure to shocks and recovery (Neocleous 2013). Really these discourses are two sides of the same coin, promoting an associationalist public ideology of vulnerable private citizens in need of the state to provide cohesion and help, in return for which they form civil associations which support governance through 'social capital', which renders political radicalism, solidarity and resistance to the state illegible—community action is either something the state can quite explicitly capitalise on as social reproduction and 'resilience' to shocks; or it is a threat to be controlled and suppressed.

These dominant academic and policy discourses in disaster studies and public health are being mobilised in the current crisis around COVID-19. They are important for our purposes here because they shape the policy, social and cultural context within which radical social forces like disaster anarchism and mutual aid operate. Since the rise of disaster studies in the 1950s, we have seen a growing trend for the state to rely on spontaneous community responses to compensate for its growing incapacity and indifference, and to manipulate media and social media to relay messages in the interests of repressive social control and behavioural nudging. At the same time, cybernetic capitalism with underpinnings in behavioural psychology has sought to securitise, quantify, privatise and scenario-build disaster response through a model that increasingly relies on an authoritarian and technocratic global policy-field (Hannigan 2012). This is incredibly profitable for private financial, development and insurance agencies (Klein 2007) but violently disempowering and dispossessive of grassroots democratic forces and movements (Solnit 2010). These dynamics reduce the capacity for social insurrection or revolution and can have a de-radicalising effect on social movements. At the forefront of the anti-authoritarian resistance, we have seen the rise of a widespread international preparedness movement drawing on mutual aid, affinity, solidarity and associated anarchist and autonomist concepts, in particular a proliferation of self-defined 'mutual aid' disaster relief movements. However, as we have already seen, state-centred discourse tends to treat people cooperating for mutual aid as a convenient source of energy to marshal temporarily for community relief action, in the interests of returning to the more 'normal' state of competitive individualism and the functioning circulation of capital. Forms of behavioural nudging are reinforced in media and social media, which many non-radical citizens are inclined to accept. The anarchist Gustav Landauer argued that the state is not only an external state of oppression, but also 'a condition, a certain relationship between human beings, a mode of behaviour; we destroy it by contracting other relationships' (Landauer 1911: 141). The middle classes and more privileged sections of society are more likely to embody the logic of the state and to act as agents of the state because they stand to benefit more, they are less likely to need mutual aid from others, and also because the kinds of 'classed practices' discussed in Chap. 3 endow them with more rigid character structures that compel them to separate from and attempt to dominate those perceived as less civilised (Reich 1911; Cudworth and Hobden 2018). In the following sections, I will consider various ways in which anarchists respond to and resist this game-rigging by attempting to situate mutual aid in a wider structural critique of capitalism and resistance to securitisation and social control.

Mutual Aid in Anarchist Theory

Mutual aid is a radical concept with a long history in the anarchist tradition of thought and practice, and is particularly associated with the work of Peter Kropotkin. A vital focus of anarchist theory is the ability to distinguish between authoritarian and anti- or non-authoritarian forms of life. In his seminal treatise on the historical rise of the state, Kropotkin (1897) argues that both reformists and revolutionaries (including Marxists and other vanguardist radicals) seeking to seize state powers are misguided, because the very essence of the state hinders the possibility of equal and free society. It is the 'extinction of local life', the seizure of local institutions for the benefit of dominant minorities, the imposition of servitude before the law and conformity of social roles within institutions. During the process of the rise of the state (which Kropotkin, similar to contemporary world systems analyst Immanuel Wallerstein, situates in the Middle Ages) people are deprived of liberties, and obliged to forget social ties based on free agreement in favour of a system where the state alone is legitimised to create union between subjects. All relationships are mediated by the 'triple alliance' of state, church and military which take on a monopoly in the task of 'watching over the industrial commercial, judicial, artistic, emotional interests' (Kropotkin 1897: 33) for which people used to unite directly. The state demands from each subject 'a direct, personal submission without intermediaries' (Ibid: 48). The political principle is 'the principle that destroys everything' and in the end, 'it is death' (Ibid: 49–59). The state is a technology of transcendental control, measurement and unification which treats people and knowledges as commensurable, therefore exchangeable, and thus creates the conditions for capitalist inequality. This account of the rise of the state as a violent process of dispossession, enclosure and destruction of communal folk knowledge in the interests of transcendental control and commensurability has been echoed and developed from feminist and postcolonial standpoints (Federici 2004; Mies 1986). The perspective of state and capital is linked to the objectification of nature as a machine rather than an organism, in a root metaphor that sanctions domination: of women, workers, animals and the environment (Merchant 1980). Similarly, open and autonomous Marxists (e.g. Hardt and Antonio Negri 2001; De Angelis 2007) and World Systems analysts (Wallerstein 2004; Amin 1990) view the state as an essentially irredeemable form of capital, or a particular alienated form of social life which reifies the political just like any other commodity and has functions which serve the interests of capital.

This literature overlaps with anarchist, eco-anarchist and communalist critiques that welfare creates dependencies which support consumerism, and deny autonomy and self-determination. Unlike classical Marxists who believe forces of production determine all other relations including the state, anarchists, open and autonomous Marxists focus on the dual role of state and capital as linked agents of alienation, with national governments supporting market expansion through colonisation and extractivism in order to secure political domination—requiring a dyadic vertical relation to the state and decomposition of horizontal social associations: people, their environments and their time become commensurable objects. The state permits people to relate only through its own mediation, which organises the people through division of labour to meet the needs of the market. In planning and preparedness, the idea that a transcendental or 'god's-eye' view is essential for coordinated action has been central to modernist democratic and technocratic projects. Standardised rules and data make local conditions 'legible' to agencies of control, but they remove control from people, which devalues local knowledge and disempowers grassroots agency (Scott 1998).

Mutual aid is the practical and economic expression of the social principle. It involves 'solidarity not charity' and seeks social change through direct action rather than reform (Spade 2020). Rather than the alienated transactional relationship assumed between professional NGO workers and 'victim', 'survivor', 'client' or 'served' communities, mutual aid presumes an equal footing—a shared empathy and humanity that means each party benefits from the relationship based on a reciprocal gift exchange (Mauss 1925). The practice aims to prefigure new affective lifeworlds by recomposing social bonds and community rather than reproducing commodified power relationships whilst creating self-management and autonomy by meeting needs directly. In anarchist theory, mutual aid is a highly politicised phenomenon which links the pleasure and joy of non-hierarchical relationships with structural critiques of capitalism and the state, by illustrating that another world is possible, and practicing it in the here-and-now. While the idea of mutual aid has been applied and advocated within everyday life by anarchists for more than a century, the idea comes into its own in the context of disasters—and in the contemporary risk-addled and disaster-prone zeitgeist, mutual aid groups are popping up at an innumerable rate. Anarchists tend to see capitalism as a disaster anyway—and mutual aid is a small-scale, everyday practice that anyone can take part in, which alleviates problems directly whilst also drawing attention to the ways in which disasters ranging from climate-related extreme weather events to biological disease tend to impact unequally on the most oppressed groups in society, who are frequently left to fend for themselves by the state. Proponents of direct-action refuse to separate means from ends and insist that we do not have to wait until tomorrow, or for state recognition, to start improving the world. Mutual aid is a prefigurative and political practice which involves helping ourselves and others directly by creating a new society in the shell of the old (Ward 1973; Gordon 2009).

Mutual Aid Disaster Relief

The first major anarchist-inspired relief efforts to hit the headlines were in the United States, including Common Ground Collective after Hurricane Katrina hit New Orleans in 2005 (crow 2014) and Occupy Sandy which assisted victims of Hurricane Sandy, which hit northeast United States in October 2012 (Firth forthcoming; Bondesson 2017). Mutual aid was happening in communities anyway, but Occupy Sandy drew upon the volunteers, latent skills, networks and platforms of the erstwhile Occupy Wall Street movement to mobilise an incredibly effective relief effort and provided an organisational infrastructure and a way for volunteers who were not already members of existing communities to join the effort. Occupy Sandy illustrated in practice that self-organised networks with low bureaucracy create faster and easier connections than bureaucratic organisations, giving them greater speed, flexibility and connectedness. They also effectively mobilised internet technology and social media, such as Google Docs, Facebook and Twitter to spread news, garner donations and mobilise volunteers, as well as using the Amazon 'gift list' facility, usually used for wedding gifts, to mobilise donations of essential items such as blankets and torches from donors worldwide (Garber 2012). Occupy Sandy was widely acknowledged even in mainstream media to have organised relief more effectively than federal agencies or NGOs (Cornish et al. 2014; Marom 2012). Conversely, the official state- and NGO-led effort following Sandy was widely perceived as a failure and produced public anger. Donor agendas led to burdensome bureaucratic requirements which impeded effective projects (Halbfinger 2012). In short, mutual aid is not only an authentic and pleasurable way of relating, it can also be a highly efficient way of providing relief in emergency situations, even in conventional terms.

Since Occupy Sandy in 2012, decentralised, anarchist-inspired mutual aid disaster relief efforts have arisen after nearly every major hurricane in the United States (e.g. Anon 2020a) and recently in the United States, longer-term preparedness networks, such as Mutual Aid Disaster Relief, have started to form, offering ongoing communications platforms, skill-shares and training (Mutual Aid Disaster Relief 2020).

Anarchist-inspired, autonomous and non-hierarchical movements have also mobilised disaster relief efforts in other countries, for example the self-managed autonomous brigades in Mexico after 2017 earthquakes (Anon 2019), grassroots village solidarity networks in Indonesia after the 2004 tsunamis (Jon and Purcell 2018), anarchist responses to Typhoon Yolanda in the Philippines in 2013 (Anon 2013, 2014) and self-management and direct action against the militarisation of disaster zones after earthquakes in Italy in 2012 and 2009 (Anon 2012a, b).

It is important to note that mutual aid is two things at once. Mutual aid is something that happens in communities anyway—during disasters and during the ongoing disaster of capitalism. It has particular roots in black and working-class communities, however they may not always choose to term it 'mutual aid' (Zuri 2020). 'Mutual aid' is thus an epistemological concept that can be used to understand a social phenomenon that would exist aside from what anarchists and other radicals decide to call it. In anarchist theory, 'mutual aid' is also a normative concept—it is something to be valued, nurtured, furthered, supported and promoted by anarchists as a fundamental part of their ideology. This phenomenon has been labelled, politicised and valorised in other ways too, for example in the United States The Black Panther Party often used the terminology of 'community social programmes', which led to a somewhat different emphasis to anarchism, particularly on the racialised aspects of oppression and exclusion, but has not prevented former Black Panther members forming projects in solidarity and alliance with anarchists, such as the Common Ground Collective hurricane relief movement after Katrina in 2005 (crow 2014). Similarly, autonomists have tended to emphasise the classed aspects of oppression and autonomy from capitalism, but in practice many projects and solidarities exist with anarchists. Anarchists are against all forms of authoritarianism and domination, including racism and classism so their ideology works well with other anti-authoritarian movements. There is a common trope, recently repeated by Donald Trump in reference to the Black Lives Matter movement, that anarchists appropriate black and working-class movements, or they are 'outside agitators' who bring violence to protests. This trope serves to undermine historical solidarities between these movements, falsely stereotypes anarchist movements as predominantly white and middle class and acts as a form of erasure of the existence of many black and working-class anarchists (Beauchamp 2020). It also serves to undermine the ways in which violence in protests and riots is often secondary, stemming from police repression of communities trying to meet their own needs through mutual aid (Robinson and Starodub 2018: 261). Therefore, while mutual aid is an incredibly effective and practical resource, it is also a radical concept and is linked to a wide-ranging critique of capitalism, racism, patriarchy and ecological domination in anarchist movements. In the following sections I will consider some of the reactions by anarchists to the COVID-19 crisis.

Mutual Aid and COVID-19

In many ways, the COVID-19 crisis and the anarchist response are similar to previous mobilisations around disasters. Similarly to environmental disasters, the communities most likely to need mutual aid are those that are hit hardest by the pandemic. In disaster research, communities identified as 'vulnerable' are those with longstanding patterns of poverty and deprivation, caused by structural factors such as inequality and austerity. Existing patterns of discrimination such as race, gender and class are likely to render people more vulnerable to a pandemic, just as they would to an earthquake or hurricane. Mutual aid tends to occur through a collaboration of radical activists who have been involved in previous actions, alongside spontaneous action that arises in communities. As a longstanding movement, current anarchist actions and projects are tied to a shared history and political culture and mobilise pre-existing networks of activists and resources. There may even be considerable overlap of people involved. This means that similar political language, organising models, skills and technologies are used, drawing on the knowledge and experience of those involved.

However, the current crisis also presents a very different context, and as such some challenges to conventional anarchist organising and models of mutual aid. COVID-19 represents an entirely new and different kind of disaster and threat to others experienced within most Western anarchists' lifetimes. In the past, mutual aid and prefigurative anarchist actions

have tended to encourage face-to-face meetings and action and have con-
flated physical and social closeness (Firth 2012). The current context
presents the challenge of an invisible contagious virus, which although it
might impact more heavily on vulnerable people at a population level,
potentially affects everyone, and can also be spread by everyone. This
forms the basis of various 'social distancing' policies and recommendations put in place by governments and other institutions to reduce the
spread of the virus through close physical contact. These measures range
from the wearing of medical or home-made masks, to standing two
metres apart from other people in public, reducing time spent outside the
house, avoiding meeting or visiting relatives or friends from other households, and in some countries there has been a need for official documen-
tation in order to leave one's own home. Not all anarchists are on board
with all of the recommendations, and critiques will be considered in
more detail below. However, a context where social distancing is backed
up by heavy policing and diffuse social pressure will have an impact on all
anarchists' activities whether they agree or not and is likely to make the
traditionally face-to-face, tactile and physical nature of mutual aid incredibly different. A pandemic also lacks the suddenness of traditional disaster work, since the agent (a virus) is much more 'complex and diffuse' and
more likely to cause chronic and long-term issues (Hannigan 2012:
13–14) requiring groups to plan and sustain action over a longer time-
frame. This slower pace affords some benefits: 'unlike terror attacks or
natural disasters, the slow burn of the pandemic allows space for critical
discussions to take place as the situation unfolds' (Donaghey 2020).

Furthermore, while there has been a growing anarchist-inspired global
movement around disasters ensuing from climate-related extreme weather
events, some parts of the world that are not usually affected by extreme
weather events or other environmental disasters, for example the UK,
have until now seen very little action related to mutual aid disaster relief.
Networks and groups are being formed and having to learn skills and
organising techniques from scratch. Unsurprisingly, while they draw on
the history of anarchist thought and practice, movements mobilising
around the pandemic have had to adapt and also exhibit some differences
to those that have previously arisen in response to weather, climate and

seismic events. This is unsurprising given the differences in context: COVID-19 is a disease, a biological phenomenon affecting human health directly, rather than an environmental phenomenon affecting humans through the more visible social mediation of infrastructure collapse—although the threat of this is also an ever-present feature of the crisis, with healthcare systems particularly at risk, alongside concerns over the supply of food and essential items. COVID-19 is much more global in its effects than even the largest scale environmental emergencies, except perhaps climate change, although in some ways this difference is redundant since anarchists tend to view local problems and political activity as interconnected and inseparable from larger structural dynamics—for example Occupy Sandy provided hurricane relief whilst raising awareness of the link between extreme weather events and climate change (Solnit 2012), and COVID-19 has shown us that the vastly unequal health outcomes between rich and poor are also connected (Solnit 2020).

At the time of writing the first draft of this chapter, just over two months since the virus emerged in China, and a matter of weeks since its spread was declared a pandemic and it arrived in my home town London, dozens of mutual aid groups had already started to spring up. At the time of editing and revising the draft, in mid-May 2020, there are more than forty groups in London, organised into hundreds of sub-groups (Freedom News 2020a), and there are over 1000 throughout the UK (Lynch and Khoo 2020). In the UK and United States, the focus of the movement appears to be a proliferation of self-described 'mutual aid' groups. These seem to have branched out well beyond customary anarchist circles and have entered mainstream consciousness. Even the American teenage magazine *Teen Vogue* has taken an anarchist stance, adopting the concept of mutual aid, and explicitly citing Kropotkin, to encourage its young readers to ensure the survival of their communities in the midst of the shortcomings and failure of political and economic systems, whilst also critiquing the authoritarian overstep of the Trump administration (Diavolo 2020).

The mutual aid movement is international and there are examples of radical action from every continent. Mutual aid groups have mobilised throughout Canada and the United States (Anon 2020b). Examples of mutual aid in the United States have included disabled activists who have produced coronavirus kits for homeless people in Oakland, California (Green 2020). Throughout the United States there are Prisoner and Migrant Detention Phone Zaps (Anon 2020b) intended to check that prisoners are being offered proper care and to overwhelm prison calling facilities with demands for increased social and healthcare rights for detainees (fight-toxic-prisons.org). Many groups have also arisen in Germany (listing.org); and there are ongoing efforts in Poland (Enough14 2020a). In Spain many grassroots organisations have arisen that were not involved in politics before, supported by the networks, knowledge and infrastructure of previous movements, including 15 M, antiracist, feminist and migrant movements (Martinez 2020). Movements have arisen in Brazil to support precarious cultural workers (Holanda and Lima 2020) and in Haiti to protect miners from exploitation (Delorus 2020). In Delhi, India, civil society actors including NGO and social workers engaged in extra-institutional direct action to resist state violence against oppressed Muslim minorities and to co-ordinate the supply of food and medicine to communities in need (Mohanty 2020). In China, examples include a group of women who have online support group for women affected by domestic violence (Bau 2020). A movement in Singapore, PinkDot, which is usually associated with protest has directed its community work inward for COVID-19, delivering care packages to LGBT activists in need (Ng 2020).

It is notable that while some of these mutual aid groups arose from pre-existing anarchist networks, others arose from non-anarchist leftist movements or from institutionalised civil society reconfiguring their actions to embrace a more direct style of action, more usually associated with anarchism, but without necessarily taking on the label of anarchist. Some, but not all, use the term 'mutual aid', and not all who use this term are anarchist, and some are unaware that the concept originates in anarchist thought. In what follows, I largely focus on the UK movement, and particularly London, where I live, and in line with the focus on the UK policy context in previous chapters. There are many parallels between the movement in London and further afield, in particular the UK and US movements seem to draw on very similar organisational models and discourse. Anarchism is a truly international movement, which does not recognise the authority of the nation state and places emphasis on local action tied to global critique. Therefore, it does not make sense to bound 'case studies' by national borders, as one might in a more conventional sociological or political analysis. Therefore, where appropriate, I have also drawn on examples from further afield to illustrate the range and variety of actions taking place. There are clearly differences in context between countries and cultures and one cannot seek to generalise too far, yet there is wider relevance and parallels with movements elsewhere.

Dean Spade (2020: 136) argues that resistant left movements model three kinds of action that directly change material conditions: '(a) work to dismantle harmful systems … (b) work to directly provide for people targeted by such systems … and (c) work to build an alternative infrastructure through which people can get their needs met'. Mutual aid addresses (b) but as has been argued above this alone is not sufficient to end capitalism and create a society without hierarchies and borders. In what follows, I will consider some of the actions that anarchists have undertaken during the COVID-19 crisis that address Spade's criteria (a) and (c), whilst adding a fourth practice, which is not often covered under the rubric of action but ought to be: (d) publishing critique—in particular, I focus on anarchist critiques of securitisation and policing in the COVID-19 crisis, and anarchist critiques of capitalism. The publishing of propaganda and critique has a long and often hidden history in anarchist movement practice (Hoyt 2014; Ferretti 2017) and it is important because it helps to raise awareness of, and identify targets for, the other modes of action. Anarchist critiques during the COVID-19 crisis have largely been online, on blogs and social media, but also through word-of-mouth and exemplary actions while engaging in mutual aid with communities.

In London, the mutual aid groups are organising a very wide range of relief and support work, generally focused around social care. There is a mutual aid group for each local borough, and these are divided by borough, zone and neighbourhood. There are also some London-wide networks and groups that co-ordinate or provide forums for people with specific interests, for example a Radical Assembly which provides a forum for radical left-wing and anarchist organisers, many of whom are dissatisfied with the lack of politicisation in their local ward. Local groups are composed of local community members helping others who are more vulnerable or who need to self-isolate to avoid spreading illness with tasks such as picking up and delivering groceries, medicines and other essentials, offering transportation to medical facilities, offering donations such as cleaning supplies, medical supplies and food for out-of-work people, offering home cooked meals, home/apartment cleaning, offering phone-calls, video chats and companionship, online entertainment such as yoga or dance classes, advice and advocacy navigating services, child care and pet care. Anarchists have also been involved in direct actions such as making masks, sewing scrubs and garnering donations of PPE for medical professionals. Similar to Occupy Sandy, these groups are utilising open source and internet technology, including Google docs with listing of groups, and being used by groups to organise resources, crowd-sourced lists of activities and initiatives, resource guides, webinars, slack channels, online meetups, peer-to-peer loan programmes and other forms of mutual aid emerging online and on-the-ground (Raymond 2020).

The mainstream perspective on disaster relief in general, and the coronavirus epidemic in particular, assumes that humans are selfish and competitive and are in need of a co-ordinating authority to tell them what to do. Mutual aid turns the conservative idea of the 'disaster utopia' on its head, positing that it is not a momentary suspension of division that leads communities to unite in mutual aid, but that this illustrates an alternative lifeworld that is normally hindered by the minorities in power and by media hegemonies (Solnit 2010: 8–9).

An interesting perspective on the current crisis is that Kropotkin's original treatise on mutual aid was in large partly a critique of the then-fashionable 'social Darwinism' of the anarchist's conservative contemporaries. Kropotkin's idea that co-operation helps species thrive more than competition seems ever-more relevant as an alternative perspective in the current conjecture where our Conservative government have been accused of openly Darwinist ideas of 'herd immunity' (Malnick 2020) and pursuing policy lines based around ideas of 'survival of the fittest'. Millstein defines mutual aid as 'collective care' involving 'making sure everyone can take time off work, have a home and enough food, stay hydrated and wash their hands, not feel alone or abandoned, receive health and other care' (Milstein 2020). Commentators have remarked how incredible it is that 'basic bonds of solidarity, empathy and altruism' have remained intact in the UK despite a decade of austerity and political polarisation (Quarshie 2020). Similar to Kropotkin, contemporary anarchists have linked their mutual aid to a radical structural critique of both the authoritarian nature of the state, and the unequal, competitive and exploitative nature of capitalism, for example an activist involved in co-operation Birmingham links the activities of their solidarity kitchen to a crisis of food poverty which has been ongoing since the 2008 crisis, resulting in the widespread use of foodbanks. The author-activist argues that food aid will become one of the most pressing concerns for the working class as we slip into recession again due to COVID-19. The food bank system is critiqued as a form of bureaucratic violence, since applicants are required to engage with a third-sector system who have a huge amount of control over the lives of the working class, who are required to explain their needs and justify themselves to paid professionals who act as gate-keepers for eligibility. This is seen to be part of a deliberate strategy of disempowerment of the working class enacted by both Tories and new Labour. It is argued that anarchists have a huge role to play in leading a radical counter-narrative of working-class empowerment and solidarity, and they argue that the popularity of the solidarity kitchen, providing over 150 free vegan meals a day, with demand far in excess of this, pays testament to the need for a political project to combat food poverty, which should operate on multiple levels: 'Both redistribution projects but also projects creating the conditions for autonomous production'. Such a project would involve not only direct provision through mutual aid, but also challenging land rights, completely re-thinking how farming and agriculture, and radically re-shaping supply chains (Yarrow Way 2020).

In the context of crises of capitalism, understanding mutual aid gets to the very heart of the nature of the relationship between state, capital and society. As described in Chap. 1, in terms of the social/political principle, the very definition of the state for anarchists is that it is parasitic of the creative energies of society. COVID-19 is exposing the fragility of capital, at the same time as capitalists are attempting to mobilise the crisis in their interests, at least partially through the technologies of the state. Radicals would argue that mutual aid and associated social responses to the pandemic are forms of social recomposition that are essentially in conflict with state and capital. The state/capital formation has at its disposal a repertoire of actions at its disposal for dealing with mutual aid, ranging from securitised and militarised lockdown rules effectively preventing the possibility of mutual aid; to a more laissez-faire neoliberal approach backed up by economic stimulus which might encourage mutual aid to flourish. From the anarchist view both stimulus and securitisation are two sides of the same coin designed to protect the needs of capital by stopping people from revolting in insurrection and/or engaging in exodus from the system by meeting their own needs though social recomposition. However, the controversy rests in the extent to which mutual aid is a radical practice that acts *against* these state-capital formations, rather than being benign or even complicit in supporting them, filling in gaps and mitigating failures. Mutual aid is in fact very convenient for governments and capitalists alike, because it creates social support systems reliant on free volunteer time, where state services are withdrawn—allowing for social and labour reproduction to continue in the midst of austerity, tax cuts for the rich and the decimation of public services. In the UK, this was even quite openly articulated as conservative policy, in the terms of David Cameron's 'Big Society' vision (Quarshie 2020) and has become part of the neoliberal, decentralising consensus. Assuming that authentic anti-authoritarian desire is possible, the political and discursive context has implications for how disaster anarchists and other radicals might seek to act during the COVID-19 pandemic.

This 'social capital' trope reappears in the liberal-Left media on COVID-19, for example Raymond (2020) rehearses phraseology of 'vulnerability' (the assumption that it is communities that are fragile, not capitalism) and 'resilience' (the idea that it is the responsibility of lower-level communities to recover from higher-level shocks, inflicted upon them by the policies of states and inequalities of capitalism—with emphasis on recovery rather than resistance or transformation). From this perspective, mutual aid is not radical, but rather creates temporary 'lifelines' for 'when government falls short', yet ultimately mutual aid is complicit with the state insofar as it has the function of restoring the normal running of things—even if the author would rather have a somewhat more social democratic, rather than neoliberal state. Rather than seeking resistance to a destructive and authoritarian complicity between state and capital, Raymond proclaims that 'it's unfortunate that those in power are unwilling to step up adequately' (Raymond 2020). From the perspective of reformist social democratic and left-liberal approaches, local movements are lauded insofar as they embody flexible and responsive local knowledge—but at the same time there is a contradictory desire to control them. Associationalist views can often come across as quite critical—for example Naomi Klein is able to critique the dispossession of communities by disaster capitalists using shock doctrine neoliberalism; yet her alternatives rely on Keynesian economic stimulus and the co-optation of social movements into a state-led social democratic consensus (Klein 2007). Anarchists and other radicals might argue that all state responses are two sides to the same coin—the choice whether to co-opt through economic stimulus and capture movements or control/repress through securitisation is always there.

The state has tried to control previous anarchist movements and community responses to disasters through severe repression. For example, after Hurricane Katrina, John Clark lists forms of oppression ranging from covert or structural violence to outright police brutality, unfair evictions, denial of prisoners' rights, de facto ethnic cleansing, mistreatment and exploitation of migrant labour (Clark 2013: 206; see also crow 2014). There has also been evidence of repression against anarchists already in the COVID-19 crisis, for example the eviction of the 'Pie 'n' Mash Squat Café' in London, which was at the time attempting to reorganise as a donation and distribution mutual aid centre. It was evicted despite the space being some people's homes, some of whom claimed to be attempting to self-isolate for public safety (Freedom News 2020b). Making people homeless during a pandemic where people are being told to 'stay at home' seems a particularly ferocious act of repression.

The state has also tried to depoliticise and de-radicalise movements through co-optation into existing organised state and institutional forms; for example claiming that mutual aid movements are apolitical and are compatible with state efforts and revising policies to attempt to incorporate them into official efforts. During Occupy Sandy, the department for Homeland Security heavily surveilled the movement, as shown in my forthcoming research, activists said they were aware of state agent surveillance and derailing of meetings during the relief process (Firth forth-coming; Smith 2014). The US Department of Homeland Security later wrote a report recommending that the actions of grassroots movements are integrated into a 'Whole Community Response', involving funding, insti-tutionalisation and bureaucratic control of movements (Ambinder et al. 2013). This is against the very spirit of mutual aid, which is characterised by anti-authoritarian horizontal organising, anti-bureaucracy and recipro-cal help—meaning no formal separation between helpers and helped. While some people may be stronger or more privileged in certain situations and therefore appear to be providing more help, the premise is that they might expect help in return if they were in a similar situation of need, and that they belong to the community that they are contributing to, rather than belonging to an alienated class of professional charity workers.

There is already evidence that state workers, professional bureaucrats and party politicians are trying to co-opt and de-radicalise mutual aid efforts in London. One activist writes of their decision to disengage with the St Peter's Ward COVID-19 mutual aid group due to a takeover by 'councillors, ex-councillors, higher-ups in NGOs and Labour Party organisers'. The author did not believe their actions to be ill-intentioned, but argued they showed a 'deliberate and wilful disregard for the basic principles of mutual aid'. This involved actions such as locking WhatsApp groups to new members, insisting on leading decisions about dividing up coverage areas (citing experience of canvassing for elections), insisting on formal leadership structures with no democratic process, holding up decisions and shutting down conversations about organisational struc-ture. Discussions about potentially more confrontational radical actions such as eviction resistance and rent striking were derailed and shut down, and there was a discussion of working with the council, including having requests for help administered through the council for 'safeguarding' rea-sons and insisting that volunteers are DBS checked. When the activist tried to remind the group of the principles of grassroots mutual aid, they were accused of 'politicising' a situation during a time when people should come together to help, however as they quite rightly argue in the article 'a mutual aid network during a time of crisis is already highly political…The liberal left has always tried to deflect criticism by accusing others of being inappropriately political, but this is only because their mode of politics is what they see as "normal", and therefore not political' (Rogers 2020).

Another activist raises similar concerns based on their experience of local councillors from the Labour Party purposefully trying to sabotage the mutual aid networks. The activist claims to have observed the same dynamics across many different groups throughout London and the UK more generally and observes that the form of disruption is similar in each case: 'a local councillor joins a locally organised WhatsApp group and begins to post confusing and/or condescending messages discouraging self-organised action, and trying to assert council control' (Spender 2020). The criticisms and derailing of autonomous action usually revolve around issues of safeguarding, including the obvious problems of using open access spreadsheets to organise deliveries to individuals' addresses who may not want their information to be in the public domain, amongst other issues. However, the 'officials' are ignoring the fact that grassroots activist groups are already providing information, training sessions and resources on this issue (see e.g. COVID-19 Mutual Aid UK 2020). Spender provides a screenshot of a conversation where the councillor attempts to talk from a position of authority about how the energy of the grassroots movement needs to be 'captured and managed in a responsible way' (Spender 2020) illustrating explicitly and vividly the way in which the logic of the state inserts itself into the self-organised affairs of ordinary people and attempts to co-opt, mediate and alienate their energies. Indeed, it appears that the UK government has incorporated the expectation of people providing mutual aid in their communities into its official social care policy for 'extremely vulnerable' people who have been told to undertake an extreme form of social isolation called 'shielding' and are informed that they can have their needs met by taking personal responsibility for reaching out to 'community groups':

> Ask family, friends and neighbours to support you and use online services. If this is not possible, then the public sector, business, charities, and the general public are gearing up to help those advised to stay at home. Please discuss your daily needs during this period of staying at home with carers, family, friends, neighbours or local community groups to see how they can support you. (Public Health England 2020)

It is not only the state which anarchists fear inserting itself into their affairs in an attempt to co-opt and de-radicalise their activities. Another anarchist from Birmingham cites 'public shitty bad-mouthing' from a cohort of Labour party members and representatives, including not only local councillors in official roles, but also a well-meaning but ultimately reformist middle class whose sense of entitlement prompts them to attempt to lead working-class movements in pursuit of selfish careerist goals and self-promotion, and through a sense nurtured by privilege that working-class movements cannot organise themselves (Anon 2020c).

The vanguardist assumption that working-class movements need outside leaders hails not only from reformist positions. It is a common trope within some forms of classical Marxism along with the Lacanian post-Marxist Left to criticise anarchist mutual aid projects for mimicking the organisational forms of capital—for example, anarchist networks are argued to mirror and to be easily (or always already) co-opted within the supposedly networked and decentralised structures of neoliberalism (e.g. Harvey 2000). Alternatively, they are too disorganised, local and particular to effect real change and deal with global problems in the absence of a centralised global authority (e.g. Zizek 2020). Ostensibly radical theorists have argued that mutual aid projects simply compensate for the austerity and withdrawal of the welfare state by performing relief work for free, and risk reproducing ideology and buttressing the interests of the wealthy and corporate sector (Chomsky 2013; Illner 2018). From these perspectives, the co-optation and de-radicalisation of anarchist mutual aid projects into the logic of the neoliberal state are no surprise. These thinkers call for anarchists to take a more politically conscious approach and allow themselves to be led by vanguards, or otherwise to form strategic coalitions.

Many anarchist activists and academics have disputed the complicity of anarchists and mutual aid in neoliberalism. Jon Bigger argues that providing social care for elderly neighbours is radical and revolutionary, because it may involve saving the lives of people that Tories don't care about (Bigger 2020). Rather than reproducing capitalism, mutual aid rather tends to reproduce life—potentially radical life—that is either disposable or a burden to capitalism. Whilst it may compensate for the withdrawal of the state, this does not mean that the state would step in in the absence of mutual aid groups, rather, people, mostly working class or otherwise marginalised, would simply suffer and die. An anonymous activist author decries co-optation by middle-class Labour voters, arguing that the very success of mutual aid lies in reaching huge swathes of vulnerable people, creating an incredible community-led safety net, and showing 'ourselves, the general public and even actual Labour voters that we don't need parties or states. We don't need anyone' (Anon 2020c). In order to understand the radicalism of anarchist mutual aid, it is important to consider it as part of a much wider repertoire of anarchist action, which sometimes brings anarchists into direct conflict with state agencies. At the same time, it is important to note that while the term 'mutual aid' derives from anarchist theory, many activists in the current conjecture see themselves neither as part of an elite vanguard, nor as part of a broader anarchist movement, but merely as normal people helping their communities—as such, they are probably better understood in Colin Ward's terms as 'anarchy in action' (Ward 1973). Nonetheless, the links to more confrontational forms of action help to refute arguments that mutual aid reproduces neoliberal austerity, allowing consideration of how anarchist theory might inform actions to resist the de-radicalisation of mutual aid.

Anarchist Actions Beyond Mutual Aid

Anarchists have called for mutual aid networks to engage in radical actions beyond simply providing food and care, particularly in actions that might be understood as forms of strike, refusal and protest or insurrection, potentially speaking to all three of Spade's criteria of (a) dismantle, (b) provide directly and (c) create infrastructure. This has included mobilising against repression to defend the homes and lives of those facing eviction, whilst also opening up empty buildings through squatting in order to provide safe spaces for homeless people to shelter and self-isolate. These actions are similar to mutual aid insofar as they follow the anarchist ethos of 'ask nothing, demand nothing' yet with the added concomitant to 'occupy and resist' these actions involve seizing 'property' and therefore bring anarchists into a much more direct confrontation with capital (F. 2020). In the UK, most actions in this category relate to occupying property and rent strikes. For example, informal unions have called for new members to join to support rent strikes during the pandemic, when many precarious workers are left unable to pay rent (London Renters Union 2020). On Mayday, squatters from across the UK co-ordinated a series of decentralised actions to highlight their plight and to address their needs—actions included occupying commercial and residential buildings, banner-drops in support of squatters facing eviction, occupying land to repurpose as open public space and to grow food (The Resi-Rectors 2020). Casting an eye on international examples, one finds a wider array of actions. Examples include students in Ohio and Massachusetts collectively rioting against police and occupied buildings when evicted from their accommodation, as some had no idea where they would go (Anon 2020d, e). Anarchists have been vocal in their support for wildcat strikes, 'sick-outs' and job actions in response to being forced to work (Anon 2020f), including workers expected to continue when one of their assembly-line co-workers already had to quarantine (Jones 2020). Anarchists have also expressed support for inmates in 30 Italian prisons who rioted and revolted—including many who escaped, and anarchist publications have translated reports from the frontlines of these struggles that otherwise would have not been covered in English-speaking media (Anon 2020g), whilst anarchists have also brought attention to prisoners' hunger strikes (Anon 2020f). Another form of refusal acts against surveillance and identification, and anarchists have raised the possibility that the normalisation of mask-wearing may raise possibilities for anonymity and a feeling of security leading to an increased ability to act in public in 'covert and cheerful situations' (Round Robin 2020). Indeed, the current scientific advice that even non-medical masks are to a degree effective in preventing spread of the virus has brought to the surface the conflict between the state's duty to protect its citizens, and its desire to repress and control them—exemplified during German Mayday protests, where the wearing of masks is illegal (Oltermann 2020).

The anarchist tradition also overlaps with and in some cases encompasses the social ecology and degrowth traditions, who have a future-oriented vision of decentralising but federated organisations and sustainable technologies, yet seeking action through mobilising groups and forces in the present (Bookchin 1971). This intellectual tradition has a practical aspect, including longer-term, committed projects such as intentional communities, eco-villages, co-operatives permaculture and transition towns. These speak to Spade's third criterion, (c), on building alternative infrastructure. Similar to the broader anarchist movement, these groups aim to inspire and extol action that takes place in the here-and-now, by ordinary people in grassroots communities and movements, rather than deferring to transcendental authorities or vanguards, or to utopias that can only occur in the future, through means which contradict their ends. Groups in this tradition have connected their mutual aid practices with prefiguration and awareness practices towards community self-sufficiency, commoning and human self-determination (Anon 2020g). Examples include a self-governed food system in Italy, CampiAperti, where farmers using sustainable agri-ecological methods and a local participatory guarantee system exchange food through networks of trust, social networks and knowledge exchange. This decentralised self-managed system has come into its own during the COVID-19 crisis, when traditional food supply chains have become insecure (Diesner 2020). Similar projects have arisen in Spanish Basque country as part of an international network (URGENCI 2020). Renowned names in the degrowth movement have argued for the nurturing of nature and people within similar projects for 'care-full degrowth' that does not glorify the temporary decline in fossil fuel and energy usage provoked by the crisis with its attendant trauma, death and impoverishment (as have some factions of the environmental Left-media), but seeks to voluntarily slow down global use of material and energy by reorienting values, institutions and worldviews. The authors recount a range of longer-term projects which are advancing degrowth via everyday practices, communal initiatives and scholarly theory (Paulson et al. 2020).

Mutual aid is itself a commoning project: a form of social recomposition whereby activists form bonds that lead to longer-term projects towards living without a state. At the same time, many mutual aid networks arise out of longer-term projects, that are often invisibilised due to the hidden nature of social movement heritage and histories: anarchist and ecological networks do not appear from nowhere nor do they fade to oblivion when the disaster is over (crow 2014: 209). While nearly all anarchist groups tend to be of a fluid and changing nature, specific crises do sometimes spawn longstanding projects, and one would expect the same from COVID-19. Some of these are likely to be absorbed into the capitalist NGO-industrial complex through a process of co-optation and bureaucratisation. While there are frequent appeals from centrists to anarchists not to politicise disaster relief, it is more often the case that powerful donors or agencies may politicise disasters by highlighting the failings of the recipient, and attaching conditions to funding (Hannigan 2012). I would predict that this will be the fate of some—but not all—of the local mutual aid groups. Alternatively, anarchist projects often endure as freestanding autonomous projects, social centres or co-operatives. There is already a thriving street medic movement in the United States (perhaps due to the ongoing disaster of their healthcare system!), which has a philosophy with roots in anarchist theory (Medic Wiki 2020). One might predict that the emerging mutual aid movement in the UK and Europe might give rise to a similar grassroots healthcare movement, given that public health systems are being decimated through austerity. While it is too early to predict how social movements emerging around the COVID-19 pandemic might crystallise into longer-term self-sufficiency projects, previous disaster anarchist movements have tended to evolve into projects involving the commoning and repurposing of space, for example in community and permaculture gardens, workers' co-operatives, intentional communities, autonomous social centres. Anarchist academic and writer Jon Bigger argues that 'the mutual aid groups springing up have to be the start, not the end. The ongoing project has to be to build real communities back up with people looking after each other beyond this virus … Society can flourish without interference from government' (Bigger 2020). There is an important emphasis on small-scale communities, which prevents people from becoming too alienated from nature and from each other, and reduces the population over which any one person or group might dominate, and the territory from which anyone can appropriate and accumulate. To understand the radical nature of the anarchist movement—and its practical instantiation in mutual aid—in the context of the COVID-19 crisis, one might also pay attention to some of the structural critiques written by anarchists, in which they often link local action like mutual aid to a much more global understanding of the operations of power—anarchism aims to destroy authoritarian power and capitalist inequality by re-scaling community, refuting the idea that mutual aid simply exists to 'fill gaps'.

Anarchist Critiques of Statist and Capitalist Disaster Response

Anarchism can be viewed as a form of disaster preparedness as it emerges from, draws on and builds the pre-existing networks, skills and volunteers of anarchist and associated non-hierarchical and anti-authoritarian leftist movements. At the same time, anarchists do not presume the same separation between different stages of disaster relief such as preparedness, response, relief and recovery—because rather than viewing disasters as a rupture in the normal running of things which should be remediated in linear fashion as soon as possible, anarchists understand disasters to be constitutive to capitalism—so a return to the normal running of things is not really desirable. Although not explicitly anarchist, Walter Benjamin's (1940) *Theses on the Philosophy of History* offers an excellent critique of idea of progress, to which capitalists and historical materialists alike are committed. He argues that in capitalism, 'state of emergency' is not the exception but the rule. Mainstream discourse on 'natural disasters' aims to depoliticise disasters as unavoidable ruptures in the normal running of capitalist progress. Therefore, conventional disaster relief tends to rest on restoring the normal running of capitalism, often claiming progress and improvement through 'development' even where this frequently means dispossessing huge swathes of communities. Anarchists have drawn attention to the importance of tying people's immediate experiences of distress and dispossession caused by emergencies to structural critiques of hierarchy and inequality.

As anti-authoritarians, anarchists are particularly aware of the dangers of state repression, securitisation and militarisation. Repressive measures adopted in a 'state of emergency' are easily absorbed into the everyday running of things, especially when backed up by the biopower of citizens in a culture of fear. Disasters are frequently heavily militarised, and policies, laws and norms put in place during a major disaster frequently do not quickly fade away (Lichfield 2020), and are adopted in adapted forms in the post-disaster society; take for instance the increased securitisation of public space and transport hubs after the terrorist attacks of 9/11, where powers the government inferred on itself were never relinquished (The South Essex Heckler 2020). Anarchists are against any increase in state power *by definition*, and the anarchist perspective views the state always and everywhere as an intrusion on self-governing and autonomous life. Anarchists believe that state claims to legitimacy are based on a fallacious view of human nature as uncooperative, selfish and oppressive. The COVID-19 crisis has given state agents even more claim to legitimacy, playing on the health fears of the population, leading to a situation where large sections of the radical Left—traditionally more allied with anarchism than the right—have been demanding stronger government—even though there is evidence that governments have already abused these powers to suspend workers' rights (Angryworkers 2020).

The cybernetic and behavioural zeitgeist has sought to securitise, quantify, privatise and scenario-build disaster response through a model that increasingly relies on an authoritarian and technocratic global policy-field (Hannigan 2012). This is incredibly profitable for private financial, development and insurance agencies (Klein 2007) but violently disempowering and dispossessive of grassroots democratic forces and movements (Solnit 2010). Nationalists and authoritarians set up a false discursive dichotomy between state-supported welfare and wellbeing programmes backed up by social control; and the vulnerabilities produced by ostensible 'freedoms' of the market. Anarchists refuse to buy into the mainstream narrative that constructs the situation as 'a trade-off between privacy and public health' (Hao 2020) or as a 'double-bind between life and freedom', for which 'we will continue paying the price long after this particular pandemic has passed' (CrimethInc 2020a). The anarchist position highlights the paradox that many non-anarchist liberals and leftists are calling for *more* repressive measures from a right-wing government that they previously criticised for its authoritarianism. Repression may also operate as internal/psychological repression, or in-group repression, or social repression (Reich 1933), for example the kinds of social pressures that are being uniformly applied to people—often by other citizens—regarding social distancing etiquette, often regardless of their particular situation. Consider the example of construction workers being judged, having been compelled to go to work, or another example of NHS workers, permitted to cycle through a park where pandemic regulations limited cycling, being abused by other park-users despite having shown their ID at the gates (Ballinger 2020). Further examples abound. This kind of civil society-based policing replicates the associationalist view of society as commensurate with 'social capital' whose purpose is ultimately to support the needs of the state and capital through cybernetic, decentralised forms of control and governance. Social democratic and left-liberal movements have united in wielding forms of biopower such as social pressure and 'blame and shame' to extol the repressive measures enacted by the state in the name of social-distancing and lockdown; a move which some anarchists have also critiqued as a worrying trend of social authoritarianism that individualises and responsibilises suffering (Round Robin 2020; CrimethInc 2020a), and acts through docile and compliant subjects who internalise state discourse, while increasing state intervention 'brings out the inner Stasi in some people' (The South Essex Heckler 2020). This dichotomy is replicated through social pressures and biopower in society, with citizens taking it upon themselves to discipline one another through managerial nudges, whilst competing selfishly for essential goods in stores. This technocratic totalitarianism, which hides behind the seemingly benign 'face of Science and Medicine, of neutrality and common interest', produces and justifies decentralised forms of authoritarianism, nurtured by structural adjustments and behavioural nudges of both states and profiteering pharmaceutical and telecommunications industries entrusted with finding a 'solution' (Anon 2020g). This will increasingly lead to cybernetic forms of governance being automated in technological surveillance through mobile devices, facial recognition and social credit systems, which have been in operation for a long time in China, South Korea and Singapore and have ostensibly proven effective in controlling citizen movements in order to track and isolate infected individuals. COVID-19 is likely to form a perfect justification for adapted forms of aggressive surveillance measures to be accelerated by Western governments (Hao 2020; Tirone et al. 2020). While cybernetic systems *appear* decentralised, they in fact rely on a totalitarian social consensus and compliance and, in the last instance, are potentially backed up with state violence. Many anarchist web articles have explicitly decried measures taken ostensibly to combat COVID-19 as authoritarian and even totalitarian, citing examples such as 'unilateral government decrees imposing total travel bans, 24-hour-a-day curfews, veritable martial law, and other dictatorial measures' (CrimethInc 2020b).

The use of the word 'totalitarian' might seem somewhat extreme from a mainstream perspective, and anarchists are often accused of being paranoid, of over-egging their critique of authority, or engaging in conspiracy theories, and in the current conjecture where conspiracy theories issuing from the Libertarian Right are rife, anarchists have seen fit to defend against such accusations. For example, one anarchist writer argues that the virus is as a convenient excuse for an economic depression that was already on the way—and an excuse to repress social movements around austerity, 'it doesn't need to be deliberate policy for it to be exploited in such a way as to exacerbate already existing separations' (Hamblin 2020). A running theme throughout the anarchist and allied anti-state Marxist response to the crisis is the identification of continuity rather than rupture between the 'normal' running of state and capitalism and the 'exceptional' circumstances of disasters. This is particularly evident in an excellent critique that expose the smooth transition and lack of clear division between democracy and authoritarianism—which from an anti-authoritarian perspective is not a digression, but 'a condition for the reproduction of the capitalist market, either at a national or even a "world system" level (Sotiropoulos and Ray 2020). Thus: The transition from a liberal democracy to an authoritarian regime (or vice versa) is usually crisis-laden, yet it still takes place within the state form which is to say, the latter absorbs the interplay between the two as moments of its own reproduction and history' (Ibid.).

As an alternative to the double-bind of the mainstream narrative, anarchists have posited the need for decentralised and un-bordered conceptions of healthcare which focus on interconnectedness and are divorced from state control (CrimethInc 2020a). Anarchist movements have therefore advocated social distancing measures with a vocabulary of co-operation, solidarity and comradeship rather than compulsion: 'Remember: that old lady you see on your grocery shopping, and that comrade you know who is suffering from a long-term illness: it is your job to protect them as much as you can'. They have similarly pointed out that inequalities mean that not everyone can easily self-isolate, for example it is particularly difficult for those in poverty and the homeless (Freedom News 2020a). Anarchists have asked for social distancing to be grounded in an ethics of care and an understanding of interconnectedness (Milstein 2020), rather than a competitive and selfish mentality reflected in governments' and technocrats' risk management programmes treating people as statistics and numbers—a discourse encouraging social competition and selfishness such as panic-buying. This ethos links to the practice of mutual aid with a supreme consistency, and furthermore, the anarchist lens might help to explain why the population under lockdown have by and large been following an ethos of protective physical distancing despite most of their interactions not being policed. It is the very premise of many seminal anarchist texts, for example Colin Ward's Anarchy in Action that most of everyday life is already anarchy, and that people do not need to be explicitly politicised as anarchists to realise that co-operation and solidarity help them to meet their needs better than competition and aggression and that individual needs are usually complimentary rather than in conflict with those of their neighbours and community (Ward 1973).

As an example of how anarchists have adapted their practices to an ethos of physical distancing, one might consider links between the mutual aid movement in some areas of London and newly occupied social centres, as part of a current revival and re-emergence of the social centres movement. Information from public websites reporting on activities shows examples of attempted co-option. For example the Green Radical Anti-capitalist Social Space (GRASS) in Islington. In February 2020 the activists found themselves in the midst of a pandemic where functioning as a traditional anarchist 'social space' was no longer viable so they responded to the virus by cancelling their events and becoming active in the local mutual aid network, transforming their space into a Mutual Aid Centre to provide a hub for community efforts. This involved storing resources needed by the network, including leaflets for outreach and disinfectant and gloves for people delivering food, as well as hosting a free clothes shop and mutual aid books donation point outside the squat and undertaking bike repairs to assist people in avoiding public transport. Whilst the activists closed the centre soon after opening in order to reduce the risk of spreading the virus, they still built and maintained good relations with the local community while following social distancing advice, raising awareness of anarchism and overcoming stereotypes about squatters and anarchists and attempting to spread the message that 'we cannot rely on the government to save us, as it will always prioritise the interests of the rich and the powerful' (GRASS 2020).

Anarchists have always been very diverse in their views, and a much smaller number of anarchists have come out against not only the police-enforced lockdown (which all anarchists must be against by definition) but have decried the near consensus with which not only Leftists, but many anarchists, have 'embraced the narrative' (Winter Oak 2020a) of social distancing. They have argued that in practice, other anarchists are not simply following a self-defined or communally decided ethos of social distancing, but rather are following the rules set by the state—a set of rules that assume the need for a co-ordinating authority, allowing the state to self-define its own legitimacy in an authoritarian power grab. Furthermore, extant social distancing rules permit 'essential' activities—defined as essential to the state, which in all cases are those which keep capitalism running—for example those that involve work and consumption, and deny the necessity of social life and protest activities essential to resistance such as gathering in public for protest.

Writers from this position have decried the tendency for the majority of anarchists to rely on 'dumbed down binary thinking' whereby they refuse to align themselves with anything tainted by the mainstream media with right-wing associations. This grouping has been keen to ally themselves with working-class insurrectionary movements like the Gilets Jaunes/Yellow Vests in France and anti-lockdown protesters in Germany. These have been accused of right-wing tendencies, yet on scrutiny defy simple divisions between right-wing and left-wing (Winter Oak 2020b; Round Robin 2020; Enough14 2020b). This position is not only taken by unknown anarchists posting anonymously online, but has been adopted also by the renowned philosopher Giorgio Agamben, who has denounced the virus as little more than a flu, and an excuse for governing powers to create a panic and institute a 'state of exception' (Agamben 2020). Similarly, another commentator predicts outbreaks of anger, resentment, protests, looting and unrest when people have enough time to think, and too little money to meet their needs—and even go so far as to encourage breaking out of quarantine to occupy public spaces, overcoming fear and risking disease in order to reinstate trust and closeness (Round Robin 2020). While this commentator's early predictions have not yet been realised and seem unlikely to come to pass, one might cite this as evidence of complicity between state and capital insofar as that the surprising initial fiscal generosity of Conservative governments has served to quell uprising. However, other anarchists have responded to this perspective, defending the need for physical/material measures to prevent the spread of the virus from a critical, anti-state perspective. They have argued against a 'deeply worrying tendency' in not only anarchism but critical theory more generally to undermine the veracity of scientific discourse 'or worse the materiality of the physical world'. However, this 'critique of the critique' also risks missing a kernel of truth concerning 'the political effects and affects of the pandemic, namely the affirmation and justification (in a substantial sense) of the state's capacity to adopt authoritarian measures and hence assume more authoritarian shapes' (Sotiropoulos and Ray 2020). Thus, some anarchists have slipped back into a depoliticised position of advocating 'tools for addressing isolation, anxiety and grief' which seem indistinguishable from a mainstream neoliberal wellbeing and resilience narrative that individualises responsibility for structural shocks without offering any practical outlet for resistance (e.g. CrimethInc 2020c; Winstanley 2020).

It is of course much easier for anarchists to remain politically active while also observing social distancing if they have a squat, social centre or commune to retreat to and use as a hub for action, just as it is often easier for middle-class members of the public to 'stay at home' than it is for the working and precarious classes. This is not to draw false equivalence between squatters and the middle class, since the former are always precarious and vulnerable to eviction, but rather to draw attention to the very wide range of structurally differentiated living conditions treated homogeneously as 'home' in public health discourse. Anarchists have been vocal critics of inequality and have critiqued scapegoating in the media and by the public of people whose housing or work precarity has prevented them from toeing the line. Again, inequality and precarity are issues of long duration that are magnified rather than caused by disasters. Repressive top-down 'public health' measures like lockdowns and surveillance are applied to all members of a population universally, despite their different vulnerabilities. These measures can make it look like the state is taking the crisis seriously, whilst covering up and compensating for decades of underfunding and attacks on healthcare services, whilst welfare concessions serve to quell uprising long enough to keep capitalism going (Anon 2020h; ACG 2020). One anarchist has pointed out that healthcare and policing have always been linked—especially evident in the use of detention, which is 'a continuation of powers which are already used regularly against Mad and Disabled people' (Evanson 2020). Anarchists have attempted to raise public consciousness by linking mutual aid activities to the fact that whilst humans are all susceptible to disease, not everyone has the same opportunities to protect or cure themselves (Anon 2020d). Anarchists have also engaged in structural and policy critique of the ways in which states and disaster capitalists might mobilise the crisis for their own interests and profits. Right-wing and (neo-)Liberal Western governments have been criticised for taking a laissez-faire approach to the health of their citizens, subordinating them to the needs of the market in a move dubbed 'herd immunity', criticised as almost a form of eugenics against older, disabled and immunocompromised people (Anarchist Federation 2020). Anarchists tend to view mutual aid and co-operation as an important constituent of 'human nature' or 'human potential' which contrasts very sharply with the conservative and new right vision of 'survival of the fittest' embedded in the idea of 'herd immunity' (Bigger 2020).

Anarchists' attention to the longue durée has led them to examine not only the ways in which capitalist exploitation is magnified by state policies around the COVID-19 virus, but also the ways in which capitalist relations are at least partly, if not wholly, to blame for the virus in the first place. Linking mutual aid to structural critique is not new—not only was it the very essence of Kropotkin's work, but one can even find a famous example linked to pandemics: in the late nineteenth century a group of anarchists including Errico Malatesta risked their lives to travel to the heart of a cholera epidemic in Naples to treat those suffering. Malateta's section had a particularly high recovery rate, which he attributed to his ability to procure food and medicine from the city authorities, and after the epidemic the anarchists published a pamphlet declaring that 'the true cause of cholera is poverty, and the true medicine to prevent its return can be nothing less than social revolution' (Fabbri 1936 cited in CrimethInc 2020d). In the current COVID crisis, one can find a version of long-term structural critique issuing from theorists thinking from the intersection of anarchism and deep ecology, which follows a similar pattern to those who seek to link specific events like hurricanes to systemic developments like climate change. While biological viruses and disease ostensibly differ drastically from environmental disasters, they also have social origins, and the ways in which disease spreads and is managed are social and environmental issues. Anarchism offers opportunities for broader critiques of where and how we live together as humans, and our relationships to animals and the natural environment. For example, renowned anthropologist James Scott has blamed human sedentism and increased drudgery during the agricultural revolution, the fragile and vulnerable nature of monocrops and reduced genetic diversity in domesticated animals for creating a perfect 'epidemiological storm' and expands this account to include 'density-dependent diseases' caused by concentration in cities and factory farming of animals (Scott 2017). An excellent article in the radical Chinese journal Chuǎng argues that mainstream perspectives try to depict COVID-19 as the eruption of wildness into civilisation, but in fact it is to do with the extension of capitalist agro-ecological value chains into previously 'wild' spheres, which changes local ecologies and modifies the interface between human and non-human (Chuǎng 2020). These arguments are not simply political or constructivist, but reflect arguments by scientists reported in mainstream media that diseases are emerging more frequently as a result of human encroachment into wild habitat (Gill 2020). Anarchist actions around this issue have included vegan collectives distributing food through mutual aid to raise awareness of the link between the spread of disease and consumption of meat (Dalton 2020).

There is a precedent in anarchist theories for thinking about long-standing and far-reaching 'wicked' problems (Cudworth and Hobden

2018: 72–3) that account for the interconnectedness of humans and nature without seeking top-down solutions. For example a 2014 article on 'An Anarchist Response to Ebola' (Bjork-James 2014a, b) which draws on the practices of non-state groups like Doctors Without Borders to envision what a wider, grassroots anarchist alternative might look like. The author argues that networks of researchers and larger frameworks of virology, medicine and epidemiology are 'among the largest decentralized efforts humans ever created', yet they are also intertwined with the modern state, echoing 'the state's urgent desire to monitor, enumerate, and plan the future of its subjects' (Bjork-James 2014b). The author envisages federated, local alternative epidemiologies that rely on federated, local-level care and multiple health organisations, involving the ongoing collection and analysis of patient data yet with secure and effective anonymisation and alongside the absence of any hierarchy of organisation; monopoly of force; and commodification of medicines or data (Ibid.). It is argued that aspects of the Ebola crisis foreshadowed such an alternative, such as community education and preparedness and the volunteer-led nature of the response in many communities. Another recent anarchist precedent which offers inspiration for thinking through 'wicked problems' is the anonymously authored pamphlet *Desert* (Anon 2011). While the author does not consider pandemics directly, the focus is on the unequal and unevenly located collapse and withdrawal of civilisation, with wealth becoming concentrated in cooler areas with some 'hot' parts of the world becoming less civilised through climate change, leading to lesser concentration of capitalism. In the process, the author argues for the resurgence of the commons in areas from which the state withdraws, including collective healthcare. There is also precedent from the British anarchist Colin Ward, who writes about de-institutionalising healthcare in an era of welfare state withdrawal (Ward 1973: 107–121). In current context of COVID-19, the flagrant flouting of lockdown rules by prime ministerial advisor Dominic Cummings has been received with shock and disdain by large sections of the British public. An anarchist might be less surprised by the blatant and disrespectful hypocrisy of an unelected technocrat, since they view hierarchical and representative government as illegitimate in the first place. Indeed one might be pleased by the prospect that public consciousness may be raised to arouse some from their Hobbesian mentality of unquestioningly following the rules because technocracy is beyond critique and the state can just confer whatever legitimacy it wants on itself in a crisis. However, the question remains: What is to be done? The flouting of the rules by the self-serving conservative elite has raised a justified fear in sections of the Left that the general populace might follow this example and risk their own families and communities' health. Anarchists would prefer rather the rules were made by communities themselves through consensus decision making or related forms of direct democracy, which included all those who stood to be affected by those rules. This would not preclude decisions informed by scientific knowledge—which might be produced and transmitted through similar models to those described in the context of Ebola, through federated organisations at different scales—for which models already exist, in the UK, for example Radical Routes and the Co-operative movement. The only obstacle we face to this vision is the current lack of infrastructure embedded in communities. Prefigurative forms of direct action such as those currently being undertaken by autonomous and anarchist movements in the UK are the most important contemporary example of such work, and the primary recommendation of this chapter would be that any reader ought—if not to join these movements themselves—to support and defend them and resist any complicity in their co-optation by the bourgeois capitalist state.

Conclusion

> I'm afraid that those who speak of oppression without acknowledging the war we are a part of, not as metaphor but as a real and current practice, will only succeed in turning a battlefield into a garden, decorating this cemetery of a society with flowers, ensuring equality of access to a graveyard. I don't care to argue that one side or another is more correct, only that revolution becomes impossible when we start believing in civil society and stop noticing that the guns are pointed at us too. (Gelderloos 2010)

The state always has the choice whether to repress mutual aid movements through securitisation or recuperate them and quell uprising through bureaucratisation, fiscal benefits and manipulating media to produce biopower. State violence and recuperation are two sides of the same coin—which come from an epistemological perspective which denies radical agency and autonomy. Right-wing populist governments such as those of the United States and UK appear to be making social democratic concessions, including stimulus packages, moratoriums on loan and mortgage interest and eviction bans, suspending arrests for minor offences; at the same time as securitising the streets through increased police presence and enforcing lockdowns, ostensibly for the public good. People are told to keep off the streets and stay in their homes, whilst vulnerable people in isolation are told to rely on deliveries and care from their 'communities' and the 'general public'. There is a mass mobilisation of biopower from leftists and liberals who were previously attacking Johnson and Trump as fascists and are now effectively urging them to be more authoritarian. Some anarchists are optimistic that the crisis might lead to positive change:

> In front of us lies the unexplored, the unknown. It is about giving up our own certainties in order to explore the infinite possibilities that await us. We will explore them with a thrill, with the excitement of discovery, with the vision of something completely new.
>
> And we will do it with joy—from the edge of the abyss, towards an uprising and liberation. (Round Robin 2020)

I am less optimistic about the possibilities that this moment will bring radical change. Disaster studies show how even though the hazards that trigger disasters might be natural, the disasters themselves are intensely social—caused by planning and infrastructure as well as the increased vulnerability of marginal populations, who are much more likely to suffer the effects of a disaster. While conspiracy theories about the virus abound, theorists of disaster capitalism, most famously Klein (2007), show how we do not need to think that disasters are man-made through a conspiracy in order to understand that powerful sociopaths will mobilise the fear, panic and momentary lack of scrutiny in their own interests. As

Lagalisse (2019) argues, the affective lack of trust expressed by many conspiracies may lead to misplaced targets, but also expresses an embryonic structural analysis that our governments may be lying to us when they imply that their foremost interest is to protect and serve us. The UK and US government policies to date seem to have been about ensuring a certain level of community transmission of the virus by keeping schools, social events and pubs open for much longer in terms of spread of the disease than other nations, while at the same time blaming their own citizens for spreading the disease while acting within the government advice and law—with government-linked advisors and officials openly speaking of 'herd immunity' to cull 'bed blockers' in hospitals (Giordano 2020). Governments are also using the virus as a premise to increase their powers, creating laws that might effectively ban some forms of political protest well beyond the duration required to deal with the pandemic. The pandemic will ensure that the rich become richer through shares in pharmaceutical companies and medical supplies. The government advice on 'protection' assumes selfish and competitive individuals, rather than mutually co-operative communities, and encourages people to fend for themselves by selfishly panic-buying, blaming and shaming perceived risky (i.e. marginalised) individuals and calling on the government to increase their already terrifying powers of control, whilst signing up for data monitoring technologies that monitor the risk of infection and seem to prefigure the kinds of oppressive social credit systems already seen in China, South Korea and Singapore.

In this chapter, I have shown how anarchists have responded by setting up mutual aid groups, engaging in acts of strike, occupation and refusal including prison breaks and riots, work walk-outs and rent strikes, setting up longer-term social centre, co-operative and food security projects. Anarchists' action is purposively local, yet their outlook is global as they engage in structural critique through their lifestyles, forms of organisation, their political culture and in their writings and publications. In the immediate term, it seems that the greatest danger for anarchists is that their radical efforts will be recuperated into the mainstream as a form of 'social capital'—or those which cannot be recuperated will be repressed through violent policing. In the longer term, anarchists must face a struggle against increasingly insidious forms of surveillance and social exclusion. Part of the argument of this chapter has been that increasingly militarised lockdowns are strengthened and not staved off by social forms of biopower, for example shaming and blaming people's behaviour in the name of promoting social distancing; or the hijacking of radical concepts by people with reformist or authoritarian desires. It is becoming clear that reformism and authoritarianism are not polar opposites as is often assumed: 'coalition politics are almost certain to end up in Popular Fronts that stifle anarchist critiques, prop up Authority, and hoodwink anti-authoritarians into being the shock troops or grunt workers for the left-wing of the system, whether in the guise of NGOs, progressive politicians, or Stalinist parties' (Gelderloos 2010). What is needed is a 'specific and foregrounded critique of recuperation' which under democratic government 'is far more common than repression as a tool for counterinsurgency' (Ibid.). This will require further theorising on how dynamics of repression and recuperation will operate in the context of the increasing automation of social control, and the production of docile and conformist subjects, through technologies such as facial recognition, social credit systems, tracking systems, privatisation and insurance of health and risk. These trends and technologies must be resisted in the hope of a more socially just and ecologically sustainable society based on ideas of mutual aid, not selfish and competitive individualism.

References

ACG. (2020). The Coronavirus Long-Term Effect. *Anarchist Communism.* https://www.anarchistcommunism.org/2020/03/24/the-coronavirus-long-term-effect/. Accessed 21 May 2020.

Agamben, G. (2020). The State of Exception Provoked by an Unmotivated Emergency. *Praxis.* http://positionswebsite.org/giorgio-agamben-the-state-of-exception-provoked-by-an-unmotivated-emergency/. Accessed 22 May 2020.

Aldrich, D. P. (2012). *Building Resilience: Social Capital in Post-disaster Recovery.* University of Chicago Press.

Alexander, J. (2020). Johnson's Message is very Deliberate and very Dangerous: Here's How to Combat It. *Medium.* https://medium.com/@jonjalex/johnsons-messageis-very-deliberate-and-very-dangerous-here-s-how-to-combat-it-d336cae96348. Accessed 13 May 2020.

Ambinder, E., Jennings, D. M., Blachman-Biatch, I., Edgemon, K., Hull, P., & Taylor, A. (2013). *The Resilient Social Network*. Department of Homeland Security Science and Technology Directorate (DHS) Publication Number: RP12-01.04.11-01.

Amin, S. (1990). *Delinking: Towards a Polycentric World*. London: Zed Books.

Anarchist Federation. (2020). More of the State You've Got (While Mutual Aid Grows to Tackle Coronavirus). *Anarchist Federation*. http://afed.org.uk/more-of-the-state-youve-got/. Accessed 19 Mar 2020.

Angryworkers. (2020). *Working Under the Corona Regime: The Current Struggles Are Taking the First Steps Towards Workers' Control*. https://angryworkersworld.wordpress.com/2020/03/24/working-under-the-corona-regime-the-current-struggles-are-taking-first-steps-towards-workers-control/. Accessed 20 May 2020.

Anon. (2011). *Desert*. Croatia: Active Distribution.

Anon. (2012a). Trieste, Italy: On the Devastation of the Rosandra Valley. *Act for Freedom*. https://actforfree.nostate.net/?p=9177. Accessed 12 May 2020.

Anon. (2012b). Earthquake in Emilia Romagna (Italy): Drones, Surveillance and Social Control. *Act For Freedom*. https://actforfree.nostate.net/?p=10073. Accessed 12 May 2020.

Anon. (2013). *Appeal from Anarchist Comrades Concerning Typhoon Yolanda (Philippines)*. https://325.nostate.net/2013/11/14/appeal-from-anarchist-comrades-concerning-typhoon-yolanda-philippines/. Accessed 12 May 2020.

Anon. (2014). *Report About Continuing Autonomous Typhoon Yolanda Disaster Relief Initiatives by Anarchists (Philippines)*. https://325.nostate.net/2014/01/03/report-about-continuing-autonomous-typhoon-yolanda-disaster-relief-initiatives-by-anarchists-philippines/. Accessed 12 May 2020.

Anon. (2019). Mexico: Political Statement from the Autonomous Brigades After the Earthquakes. *It's Going Down* (September 21, 2017). https://itsgoingdown.org/mexico-autonomous-brigades-earthquakes/. Accessed Jan 2020.

Anon. (2020a). When Flood Waters Run Dry: Hurricane Harvey, Climate Change and Social Reproduction. *It's Going Down*. https://itsgoingdown.org/when-flood-waters-run-dry-hurricane-harvey-climate-change-social-reproduction/. Accessed 12 May 2020.

Anon. (2020b). COVID-19 Mutual Aid. *It's Going Down*. https://itsgoingdown.org/c19-mutual-aid/. Accessed 22 Mar 2020.

Anon. (2020c). Mutual Aid: It's a Class Sabotage! *Freedom News*. https://freedomnews.org.uk/mutual-aid-its-a-class-sabotage/. Accessed 20 May 2020.

Anon. (2020d). 'Tear Gas Can't Stop Us': Police Fire Projectiles at Ohio Students After School Moves to Close Due to Coronavirus. https://itsgoingdown.org/tear-gas-cant-stop-us-dayton/. Accessed 20 May 2020.

Anon. (2020e). 'Warzone': MIT Students Enraged by Coronavirus Banishment. *The Daily Beast.* https://www.thedailybeast.com/warzone-mit-students-enraged-by-coronavirus-banishment. Accessed 20 May 2020.

Anon. (2020f). Workers Launch Wave of Wildcat Strikes as Trump Pushes for 'Return to Work' Amidst Exploding Coronavirus. *It's Going Down.* https://itsgoingdown.org/workers-walk-off-job-coronavirus/. Accessed 20 May 2020.

Anon. (2020g). Via Nantes Indymedia, France. The Worst Virus Ever … Authority. *325*, trans. Anarchists Worldwide. Available at: https://325.nostate.net/2020/03/16/france-the-worst-virus-ever-authority/#more-26484. Accessed 18 Mar 2020.

Anon. (2020h). The 'Scientific Rigour' Which Has Left Our Hospitals Unprepared. *Freedom News.* https://freedomnews.org.uk/the-scientific-rigour-which-has-left-our-hospitals-unprepared/. Accessed 21 May 2020.

Ballinger, A. (2020). NHS Staff 'Stopped Cycling to Work Through Richmond Park' Due to Abuse. *Cycling Weekly.* https://www.cyclingweekly.com/news/latest-news/nhs-staff-stopped-cycling-to-work-through-richmond-park-due-to-abuse-456594. Accessed 27 May 2020.

Barton, A. H. (1969). *Communities in Disaster: A Sociological Analysis of Collective Stress Situations.* New York: Doubleday.

Bau, H. (2020). 'Anti-Domestic Violence Little Vaccine': A Wuhan-Based Feminist Activist Campaign During COVID-19. *Interface: A Journal for and About Social Movements Sharing Stories of Struggles.* https://www.interface-journal.net/wp-content/uploads/2020/05/Bao.pdf. Accessed 17 May 2020.

Beauchamp, Z. (2020, June 8). Antifa, Explained: What the Left-Wing Movement Actually Believes – And Why President Trump's Scapegoating of Them During the George Floyd Protests Is so Dangerous. *Vox.* https://www.vox.com/policy-and-politics/2020/6/8/21277320/antifa-anti-fascist-explained. Accessed 9 June 2020.

Beck, U. (2002). *Risk Society: Towards a New Modernity.* New York: Sage.

Benjamin, W. (1940). *Theses on the Philosophy of History.* https://www.sfu.ca/~andrewf/CONCEPT2.html. Accessed 22 Mar 2020.

Bigger, J. (2020). Covid 19 Exposes the Evil Nature of Conservatism. *Freedom News.* https://freedomnews.org.uk/covid19-exposes-the-evil-nature-of-conservatism/. Accessed 22 Mar 2020.

Bjork-James, C. (2014a). An Anarchist Response to Ebola, Part One: What Went Wrong. *Anarchist Agency*. https://www.anarchistagency.com/commentary/an-anarchist-response-to-ebola-part-one/. Accessed 19 Mar 2020.

Bjork-James, C. (2014b). An Anarchist Response to Ebola, Part Two: Envisioning an Anarchist Alternative. *Anarchist Agency*. https://www.anarchistagency.com/commentary/an-anarchist-response-to-ebola-part-two/. Accessed 19 Mar 2020.

Boltanski, L., & Chiapello, E. (2005). The New Spirit of Capitalism. *International Journal of Politics, Culture, and Society, 18*(3–4), 161–188.

Bondesson, S. (2017). *Vulnerability and Power: Social Justice Organizing in Rockaway, New York City, After Hurricane Sandy.* PhD thesis, Uppsala University.

Bookchin, M. (1971). *Post-Scarcity Anarchism.* Berkeley: Ramparts Press.

Bruff, I. (2014). The Rise of Authoritarian Neoliberalism. *Rethinking Marxism, 26*(1), 113–129.

Chomsky, N. (2013, February 26). The Lateral State of America [Interview]. *The Occupied Times of London.* https://theoccupiedtimes.org/?p=8191. Accessed 19 Mar 2020.

Chuǎng. (2020). *Social Contagion: Microbiological Class War in China.* http://chuangcn.org/about/. Accessed 12 May 2020.

Clark, J. P. (2013). Disaster Anarchism: Hurricane Katrina and the Shock of Recognition. In J. P. Clark (Ed.), *The Impossible Community: Realizing Communitarian Anarchism* (pp. 193–216). New York: Bloomsbury Publishing USA.

Cornish, F., Montenegro, C., Reisen, K., Zaka, F., & Sevitt, J. (2014). Trust the Process: Community Health Psychology After Occupy. *Journal of health psychology, 19*(1), 60–71.

COVID-19 Mutual Aid UK. (2020). *Resources,* https://covidmutualaid.org/resources/. Accessed 20 May 2020.

CrimethInc. (2020a). *Against the Coronavirus and the Opportunism of the State: Anarchists in Italy Report on the Spread of the Virus and the Quarantine.* https://crimethinc.com/2020/03/12/against-the-coronavirus-and-the-opportunism-of-the-state-anarchists-in-italy-report-on-the-spread-of-the-virus-and-the-quarantine. Accessed 21 May 2020.

CrimethInc. (2020b). *Surviving the Virus, An Anarchist Guide: Capitalism in Crisis, Rising Totalitarianism, Strategies of Resistance.* https://crimethinc.com/2020/03/18/surviving-the-virus-an-anarchist-guide-capitalism-in-crisis-rising-totalitarianism-strategies-of-resistance. Accessed 21 May 2020.

CrimethInc. (2020c). Surviving a Pandemic: Tools for Addressing Isolation, Anxiety, and Grief. *CrimethInc.* https://crimethinc.com/2020/05/07/surviving-a-pandemic-tools-for-addressing-isolation-anxiety-and-grief. Accessed 22 May 2020.

CrimethInc. (2020d). The Anarchists Versus the Plague: Malatesta and the Cholera Epidemic of 1884. *CrimethInc.* https://crimethinc.com/2020/05/26/the-anarchists-versus-the-plague-malatesta-and-the-cholera-epidemic-of-1884#fn:1. Accessed 27 May 2020.

crow, scott. (2014). *Black Flags and Windmills: Hope, Anarchy, and the Common Ground Collective*. Oakland: PM Press. [Note: Crow Spells His Name in Lower Case].

Cudworth, E., & Hobden, S. (2018). *The Emancipatory Project of Posthumanism*. London/New York: Routledge.

Dalton, J. (2020, May 5). Vegan Group Gives Away Thousands of Means to Help the Hungry and Warns of Dangers of Animal Consumption. *The Independent*. https://www.independent.co.uk/news/uk/home-news/coronavirus-help-the-hungry-meals-vegan-animals-plant-based-london-a9497816.html. Accessed 20 May 2020.

Davis, M. (2005). *The Monster at Our Door: The Global Threat of Avian Flu*. New York: The New Press.

Davis, M. (2020). COVID-19: The Monster Is Finally at the Door. *LINKS: International Journal of Socialist Renewal*. http://links.org.au/mike-davis-covid-19-monster-finally-at-the-door?fbclid=IwAR3bgc5JA846V16MuAtFG2HDrY78BsIoWGLXkioXrUkA4fJ6oTP0AhJwjsI. Accessed 15 May 2020.

De Angelis, M. (2007). *The Beginning of History: Value Struggles and Global Capital*. London: Pluto Press.

Diavolo, L. (2020, March 16). People Are Fighting the Coronavirus with Mutual Aid Efforts to Help Each Other. *Teen Vogue*. https://www.teenvogue.com/story/people-fighting-coronavirus-mutual-aid-efforts-help-each-other?fbclid=IwAR0ZbFB5FUqj0E-losJJorgT4UYlTOCHpK1tQic24R4g1omodz0zI9GhrA0. Accessed 16 May 2020.

Diesner, D. (2020). Self-Governance Food System in Italy: Self-Governance Food System Before and During the Covid-Crisis on the Example of CampiAperti, Bologna, Italy. *Interface: A Journal for and About Social Movements*. https://www.interfacejournal.net/wp-content/uploads/2020/05/Diesner.pdf. Accessed 20 May 2020.

Donaghey, J. (2020, April 13). 'It's Going to Be Anarchy' (Fingers Crossed): Anarchist Analyses of the Coronavirus/COVID-19 Pandemic Crisis.

Anarchist Studies Blog 2020. https://anarchiststudies.noblogs.org/article-its-going-to-be-anarchy-fingers-crossed-anarchist-analyses-of-the-coronavirus-covid-19-pandemic-crisis/#_ednref1. Accessed 1 May 2020.

Drury, J., Cocking, C., & Reicher, S. (2009). The Nature of Collective Resilience: Survivor Reactions to the 2005 London Bombings. *International Journal of Mass Emergencies and Disasters, 27*(1), 66–95.

Enough14. (2020a). *#Coronavirus, #Poznan, #Poland: The State Will Disappoint You. The #COVID19 Epidemic Requires Mutual Aid.* https://enoughisenough14.org/2020/03/15/coronavirus-poznan-poland-the-state-will-dissapoint-you-the-covid19-epidemic-requires-mutual-aid/. Accessed 22 May 2020.

Enough14. (2020b). *The Emerging #Pandemic Fascism – Fragments of Dissonance.* https://enoughisenough14.org/2020/03/28/the-emerging-pandemic-fascism-fragments-of-dissonance/#comments. Accessed 22 May 2020.

Erikson, K. (1991). Notes on Trauma and Community. *American Imago, 48*(4), 455–472.

Evanson, D. (2020). Listen Up Sanes: The Intersection of Policing and Healthcare Is Nothing New. *Freedom News.* https://freedomnews.org.uk/listen-up-sanes-the-intersection-of-policing-and-healthcare-is-nothing-new/. Accessed 20 May 2020.

F., G. (2020). To the MAN: Zero Evictions Call-Out. *Freedom News.* https://freedomnews.org.uk/to-the-man-zero-evictions-call-out/. Accessed 28 October 2020.

Fabbri, L. (1936). Life of Malatesta. *Anarchy Archives.* http://dwardmac.pitzer.edu/anarchist_archives/malatesta/lifeofmalatesta.html#p116. Accessed 27 May 2020.

Federici, S. (2004). *Caliban and the Witch: Women, the Body and Primitive Accumulation.* New York: Autonomedia.

Ferretti, F. (2017). Publishing Anarchism: Pyotr Kropotkin and British Print Cultures, 1876–1917. *Journal of Historical Geography, 5717–5727.*

Fight-toxic-prisons.org. (2020). *Macomb Correctional (MI) – Coronavirus Phone Zap!* https://fight-toxic-prisons.org/2020/03/12/macomb-ci-coronavirus-phone-zap/. Accessed 17 May 2020.

Firth, R. (forthcoming). *Disaster Anarchism.* London: Pluto.

Firth, R. (2012). *Utopian Politics: Citizenship and Practice.* London: Routledge.

Franks, B. (2020). *Anarchisms, Postanarchisms and Ethics.* London: Rowman and Littlefield.

Freedom News. (2020a). *COVID-19 Mutual Aid Groups: A List.* https://freedomnews.org.uk/covid-19-uk-mutual-aid-groups-a-list/. Accessed 18 Mar 2020.

Freedom News. (2020b). London: Eviction of the Pie 'N' Mash Squat Café – We Must Push for No Evictions in This Crisis! *Freedom News*. https://freedomnews.org.uk/london-eviction-of-the-pie-n-mash-squat-cafe-we-must-push-for-no-evictions-in-this-crisis/. Accessed 22 Mar 2020.

Fritz, C. E. (1966). *Disasters and Mental Health: Therapeutic Principles Drawn from Disaster Studies*, University of Delaware Disaster Research Center.

Garber, M. (2012, November 5). Occupy Sandy Hacks Amazon's Wedding Registry (in a Good Way). *The Atlantic*. https://www.theatlantic.com/technology/archive/2012/11/occupy-sandy-hacks-amazons-wedding-registry-in-a-good-way/264543/. Accessed 14 Jan 2020.

Gelderloos, P. (2010). Lines in the Sand. *The Anarchist Library*. http://theanarchistlibrary.org/library/peter-gelderloos-lines-in-sand. Accessed 23 Mar 2020.

Gill, V. (2020). Coronavirus 'Missing Link' Species may Never be Found. *BBC News*, 4 May 2020. https://www.bbc.co.uk/news/science-environment-52529830. Acessed May 4 2020.

Giordano, C. (2020). *Coronavirus: Leading Ex-nurse says Pandemic would be 'useful' in Solving Bed Blocking by Killing off Patients*. https://www.independent.co.uk/news/health/coronavirus-news-uk-latest-june-andrews-bed-blockers-hospitals-scottish-parliament-a9384116.html. Accessed 25 March 2020.

Gordon, U. (2009). Dark Tidings: Anarchist Politics in the Age of Collapse. In R. Amster, A. DeLeon, L. A. Fernandez, A. J. Nocella II, & D. Shannon (Eds.), *Contemporary Anarchist Studies* (pp. 249–258). London: Routledge.

GRASS. (2020). Green Radical Anticapitalist Social Space. *Network 23*. https://network23.org/grass/. Accessed 21 May 2020.

Green, M. (2020). Coronavirus: How These Disabled Activists Are Taking Matters into Their Own (Sanitized) Hands. *KQED*. https://www.kqed.org/news/11806414/coronavirus-how-these-disabled-activists-are-taking-matters-into-their-own-sanitized-han?fbclid=IwAR1yyacv0WWEK3tvI2fk2r6usXSKMGgSc6E3V3O82C_kLhCQS9NTZfoMic8. Accessed 19 Mar 2020.

Halbfinger, D. M. (2012, November 12). Anger Grows at Response by Red Cross. *The New York Times*. http://www.nytimes.com/2012/11/03/nyregion/anger-grows-at-the-red-cross-response-to-the-storm.html. Accessed 12 May 2020.

Hamblin, J. (2020, January 24). A Historic Outbreak: China's Attempt to Curb a Viral Outbreak Is a Radical Experiment in Authoritarian Medicine. *The Atlantic*. https://www.theatlantic.com/health/archive/2020/01/china-quarantine-coronavirus/605455/?utm_source=HRIC+Updates&utm_campaign=b444582402-EMAIL_CAMPAIGN_2018_12_04_11_54_COPY_01&utm_medium=email&utm_term=0_b537d30fde-b444582402-259226909. Accessed 20 May 2020.

Hannigan, J. (2012). *Disasters without Borders: The International Politics of Natural Disasters.* Cambridge: Polity Press.

Hao, K. (2020, March 24). Coronavirus Is Forcing a Trade-Off Between Privacy and Public Health. *MIT Technology Review.* https://www.technologyreview.com/s/615396/coronavirus-is-forcing-a-trade-off-between-privacy-and-public-health/. Accessed 25 Mar 2020.

Hardt, M., & Antonio Negri, A. (2001). *Empire.* Cambridge, MA: Harvard University Press.

Harvey, D. (2000). *Spaces of Hope.* Berkeley: University of California Press.

Holanda, N., & Lima, V. (2020). Movimentos e ações político-culturais do Brasil em tempos de pandemia do COVID-19. *Interface: A Journal for and About Social Movements.* https://www.interfacejournal.net/wp-content/uploads/2020/05/Holanda-e-Lima.pdf. Accessed 17 May 2020.

Hoyt, A. (2014, Fall). Hidden Histories and Material Culture: The Provenance of an Anarchist Pamphlet. *Zapruder World: An International Journal for the History of Social Conflict,* Volume 1 – The Whole World Is Our Homeland: Italian Anarchist Networks in Global Context, 1870–1939, Odradek Edizioni.

Illner, P. (2018). The Locals Do It Better? The Strange Victory of Occupy Sandy. In R. Bell & R. Ficociello (Eds.), *Eco-Culture: Disaster, Narrative, Discourse.* Lanham: Lexington Books.

Jon, I., & Purcell, M. (2018). Radical Resilience: Autonomous Self-Management in Post-Disaster Recovery Planning and Practice. *Planning Theory & Practice, 19*(20), 235–251.

Jones, S. (2020). Workers Halt Production at Fiat Chrysler Windsor Assembly over Coronavirus Danger. *World Socialist Web Site.* https://www.wsws.org/en/articles/2020/03/14/shap-m14.html. Accessed 22 May 2020.

Klein, N. (2007). *The Shock Doctrine: The Rise of Disaster Capitalism.* New York: Allen Lane.

Kropotkin, P. (1897). *The State: Its Historic* Role (V. Richards, Trans. 1997). London: Freedom Press.

Lagalisse, E. (2019). *Occult Features of Anarchism: With Attention to the Conspiracy of Kings and the Conspiracy of the Peoples.* Oakland: PM Press.

Landauer, G. (1911). *For Socialism* (D. J. Parent, Trans. 1978). St. Louis: Telos Press.

Lash, S., & Urry, J. (1987). *The End of Organised Capitalism.* Cambridge: Polity.

Lichfield, G. (2020). We're Not Going Back to Normal. *MIT Technology Review.* https://www.technologyreview.com/s/615370/coronavirus-pandemic-social-distancing-18-months/?utm_source=pocket-newtab. Accessed 25 Mar 2020.

Listing.org. (2020). *Solidarische Nachbarschaftshilfe.* https://listling.org/lists/ pwfjfkpjmesjjinm/solidarische-nachbarschaftshilfe. Accessed 20 Mar 2020.

London Renters Union (2020). *Join Us.* Available from https://londonrentersunion.org/join/. Accessed 18 March 2020.

Lynch, P., & Khoo, A. (2020). Coronavirus: Volunteers Flock to Join Community Support Groups. *BBC.com.* https://www.bbc.co.uk/news/uk-england-51978388. Accessed 16 May 2020.

Malnick, E. (2020). *Government Scientists Talked Up Herd Immunity Despite Warnings of Early Reinfection.* https://www.telegraph.co.uk/news/2020/05/17/ government-scientists-talked-herd-immunity-despite-warnings/. Accessed 18 May 2020.

Marom, Y. (2012). Occupy Sandy: From Relief to Resistance. *Waging Nonviolence.* http://wagingnonviolence.org/feature/occupy-sandy-from-relief-to-resistance/. Accessed 12 May 2020.

Martinez, M. A. (2020). Mutating Mobilisations During the Pandemic Crisis in Spain. *Interface: A Journal for and About Social Movements.* https://www. interfacejournal.net/wp-content/uploads/2020/05/Martinez.pdf. Accessed 16 May 2020.

Mathbor, G. M. (2007). Enhancement of Community Preparedness for Natural Disasters: The Role of Social Work in Building Social Capital for Sustainable Disaster Relief and Management. *International Social Work, 50*(3), 357–369.

Mauss, M. (1925 [2002]). *The Gift: The Form and Reason for Exchange in Archaic Societies.* London: Routledge.

Medic Wiki. (2020). Street Medic History and Philosophy. *Medic Wiki.* https:// medic.wikia.org/wiki/Street_medic_history_and_philosophy. Accessed 20 May 2020.

Merchant, C. (1980). *The Death of Nature: Women, Nature and the Scientific Revolution.* New York: Harper and Row.

Mies, M. (1986 [2014]). *Patriarchy and Accumulation on a World Scale: Women in the International Division of Labour.* London: Zed Books.

Milstein, C. (2020). Collective Care Is Our Best Weapon Against COVID-19. *Mutual Aid Disaster Relief.* https://mutualaiddisasterrelief.org/collective-care/ ?fbclid=IwAR28tHJ3yNRyuaBUWE9sxGUgq18L6aGTOJBGj7JcVu0rfG g4UWKxzPM204I. Accessed 18 May 2020.

Mohanty, S. (2020). From Communal Violence to Lockdown Hunger: Emergency Responses by Civil Society Networks in Delhi India. *Interface: A Journal for and About Social Movements.* https://www.interfacejournal.net/ wp-content/uploads/2020/04/Mohanty.pdf. Accessed 17 May 2020.

Mutual Aid Disaster Relief. (2020). https://mutualaiddisasterrelief.org/. Accessed 19 Mar 2020.

Nakagawa, Y., & Shaw, R. (2004). Social Capital: A Missing Link to Disaster Recovery. *International Journal of Mass Emergencies and Disasters, 22*(1), 5–34.

Neocleous, M. (2013). Resisting Resilience. *Radical Philosophy, 178*(6). Available at: https://www.radicalphilosophy.com/commentary/resisting-resilience. Accessed 16 May 2020.

Ng, Lynn Ling Yu. (2020). What Does the COVID-19 Pandemic Mean for PinkDot Singapore? *Interface: A Journal for and About Social Movements.* https://www.interfacejournal.net/wp-content/uploads/2020/04/Ng.pdf. Accessed 17 May 2020.

Oliver-Smith, A. (1999). The Brotherhood of Pain: Theoretical and Applied Perspectives on Post-disaster Solidarity. *The Angry Earth: Disaster in Anthropological Perspective*, 156–172.

Oliver-Smith, A., & Hoffman, S. M. (2002). Introduction: Why Anthropologists Should Study Disasters. In S. M. Hoffman & A. Oliver-Smith (Eds.), *Catastrophe and Culture: The Anthropology of Disaster* (pp. 3–22). Santa Fe: School of American Research Press.

Oltermann, P. (2020). German Police Face Dilemma as May Day Activists Plan to Cover Faces. *The Guardian.* https://www.theguardian.com/world/2020/apr/29/mask-dilemma-for-police-in-germany-as-may-day-activists-cover-up?fbclid=IwAR3icnpUG8lQnypN1gflCKj7S38ObIDrgvaSukPKIclsnhYO YiHXJKXdgmg. Accessed 20 May 2020.

Paulson, S., D'Alisa, G., Demaria, F., & Kallis, G. with Feminisms and Degrowth Alliance. (2020). From Pandemic Toward Care-Full Degrowth. *Interface: A Journal for and About Social Movements.* https://www.interfacejournal.net/wp-content/uploads/2020/05/Paulson-et-al.pdf. Accessed 20 May 2020.

Public Health England. (2020). Guidance on Shielding and Protecting People defined on Medical Grounds as Extremely Vulnerable from COVID-19. Gov.uk, 21 March 2020. https://www.gov.uk/government/publications/guidance-on-shielding-and-protecting-extremely-vulnerable-persons-from-covid-19/guidance-onshielding-and-protecting-extremely-vulnerable-persons-from-covid-19?fbclid=IwAR22XLO6KK5ZmyA4NY_1hSBRuaXlxO0Rv6Rojb7VLJhVXFLzeTo5282a16E#what-is-the-advice-for-informal-carers-who-provide-care-forsomeone-who-is-extremely-vulnerable. Accessed 23 March 2020.

Putnam, R. (1993). *Making Democracy Work: Civic Traditions in Modern Italy.* Princeton: Princeton University Press.

Quarantelli, E. L. (1998). *Major Criteria for Judging Disaster Planning and Managing Their Applicability in Developing Countries*. University of Delaware Disaster Research Center, Preliminary Paper #268. http://udspace.udel.edu/bitstream/handle/19716/286/PP268.pdf?sequence=1&isAllowed=y. Accessed 9 July 2020.

Quarshie, A. (2020). Solidarity in Times of Crisis. *Verso books blog*. https://www.versobooks.com/blogs/4619-solidarity-in-times-of-crisis. Accessed 18 May 2020.

Raymond, R. (2020). Coronavirus Catalyses Growing Wave of Grassroots Action Despite Social Distancing. *Shareable*. https://www.shareable.net/coronaviruscatalyzes-growing-wave-of-grassroots-action-despite-social-distancing/. Accessed 20 March 2020.

Reich, W. (1911). *Character Analysis*. 3rd ed., 1980. New York: Macmillan.

Reich, W. (1933). *The Mass Psychology of Fascism* (V. R. Carfagno, Trans. 1970). London: Penguin Books.

Robinson, A., & Starodub, A. (2018). Conclusion: Some Reflections on Contemporary Riots and Militant Occupations. In Starodub, A. And Robinson, A. (Ed.), *Riots and Militant Occupations: Smashing a System, Building a World – A Critical Introduction* (pp. 257–252). London: Rowman and Littlefield.

Rogers, J. (2020). Mutual Aid in London: A Cautionary Tale. *Freedom News*. https://freedomnews.org.uk/mutual-aid-in-london-a-cautionary-tale/. Accessed 22 Mar 2020.

Round Robin. (2020). Insurrection in Times of #Coronavirus. *Enough 14*. https://enoughisenough14.org/2020/03/18/insurrection-in-times-of-the-coronavirus/. Accessed 19 Mar 2020.

Scott, J. C. (1998). *Seeing Like a State: How Certain Schemes to Improve the Human Condition Have Failed*. New Haven: Yale University Press.

Scott, J. C. (2017). *Against the Grain: A Deep History of the Earliest States*. New Haven: Yale University Press.

Smith, E. (2014). *The State, Occupy and Disaster: What Radical Movement Builders Can Learn from the Case of Occupy Sandy*. https://thetempworker.wordpress.com/2014/08/29/the-state-occupy-and-disaster-what-radical-movement-builders-can-learn-from-the-case-of-occupy-sandy/. Accessed 19 Nov 2019.

Solnit, R. (2010). *A Paradise Built in Hell: The Extraordinary Communities that Arise in Disaster*. New York: Penguin.

Solnit, R. (2012). The Name of the Hurricane Is Climate Change. *The Nation*. Available at https://www.thenation.com/article/name-hurricane-climate-change/. Accessed 16 May 2020.

Solnit, R. (2020, April 7). 'The Impossible Has Already Happened': What Coronavirus Can Teach Us About Hope. *The Guardian*. https://www.the-guardian.com/world/2020/apr/07/what-coronavirus-can-teach-us-about-hope-rebecca-solnit. Accessed 22 May 2020.

Sotiropoulos, G., & Ray, G. (2020). Pandemic Dystopias: Biopolitical Emergency and Social Resistance. *Void Network*. https://voidnetwork.gr/2020/04/04/pandemic-dystopias-biopolitical-emergency-and-social-resistance/. Accessed 20 May 2020.

Spade, D. (2020). Solidarity Not Charity: Mutual Aid for Mobilization and Survival. *Social Text, 38.1*(142), 131–151.

Spender, C. (2020). Local Councils Are Already Trying to Sabotage the Mutual Aid Networks. *Freedom News*. https://freedomnews.org.uk/local-councils-are-already-trying-to-sabotage-the-mutual-aid-networks/. Accessed 22 Mar 2020.

The Invisible Committee. (2014). *To Our Friends*. South Pasadena: semiotext(e).

The Resi-Rectors. (2020). UK: Evictions Make Us Sick! *squat.net*. https://en.squat.net/2020/05/02/uk-evictions-make-us-sick/. Accessed 20 May 2020.

The South Essex Heckler. (2020). *The COVID-19 Crisis and the Loss of Freedom*. https://thehecklersewca.wordpress.com/2020/03/30/the-covid-19-crisis-and-the-loss-of-freedom/. Accessed 20 May 2020.

Tirone, J., Seal, T., & Drozdiak, N. (2020). Location Data to Gauge Lockdowns Tests Europe's Love of Privacy. *Bloomberg.com*. https://www.bloomberg.com/news/articles/2020-03-18/austria-italy-join-push-to-use-mobile-data-to-gauge-lockdown?fbclid=IwAR0gEXMV9Sunre9v3fY_iAMlpPXNWQd5b-mIZytTnaKVCePXmOHJkHA85DwY. Accessed 25 Mar 2020.

URGENCI. (2020). Community Supported Agriculture Is a Safe and Resilient Alternative to Industrial Agriculture in the Time of COVID-19. *Interface: A Journal for and About Social Movements*. https://www.interfacejournal.net/wp-content/uploads/2020/04/URGENCI-virus-and-CSAs.pdf. Accessed 20 May 2020.

Wallerstein, I. M. (2004). *World-Systems Analysis: An Introduction*. Durham: Duke University Press.

Ward, C. (1973). *Anarchy in Action*. London: Freedom Press.

Winstanley, C. (2020). Responsibilising Corona. *Plan C*. https://www.weareplanc.org/blog/responsibilising-corona/?fbclid=IwAR1FIOpqPxytlO

WmC-2eYXeCTaHckakM9RXaMtK30IQj5yXMgq6pPrU1D0c.   Accessed 24 Mar 2020.

Winter Oak. (2020a). Anarchists and the Coronavirus. *The Acorn: An Organic Radical Bulletin*. https://winteroak.org.uk/2020/04/03/anarchists-and-the-coronavirus/. Accessed 7 May 2020.

Winter Oak. (2020b). The Acorn: Resistance Update. *The Acorn: An Organic Radical Bulletin*. https://winteroak.org.uk/2020/05/. Accessed 20 May 2020.

Wolfenstein, M. (1957). *Disaster: A Psychological Essay*. New York: Routledge.

Yarrow Way. (2020). Food, Poverty, Mutual Aid: Reflections from Birmingham Solidarity Kitchen. *Freedom News*. https://freedomnews.org.uk/food-poverty-mutual-aid-reflections-from-birmingham-solidarity-kitchen/. Accessed 19 May 2020.

Zuri, E. K. (2020). 'We've Been Organising Like This Since Day' – Why We Must Remember the Black Roots of Mutual Aid Groups. *gal-dem*. https://gal-dem.com/weve-been-organising-like-this-since-day-why-we-must-remember-the-black-roots-of-mutual-aid-groups/. Accessed 9 June 2020.

Index

© The Author(s) 2020
J. Preston, R. Firth, *Coronavirus, Class and Mutual Aid in the United Kingdom*,
https://doi.org/10.1007/978-3-030-57714-8